Praise for *Anatomy of Research for Nurses*

"Anatomy of Research for Nurses *fills an important niche. Its focus on the basics of nursing research addresses important gaps in the critically important area of evidence-based practice in an approachable, creative, and engaging manner. The authors and their colleagues are to be commended on this important work.*"

—, FAAN
School of Nursing

"*As we seek to deliver better, faster, and more affordable care for more patients, nurses are challenged as never before to provide evidence-based care. The conventional wisdom, 'Do more with less,' is not the solution. We are obligated to do only the right things and do them as cost-effectively as possible. This book guides direct-care nurses in using and generating the evidence required to achieve quality with economy, the outcome we seek for our patients and our profession.*"

—Mary Tonges, PhD, RN, NEA-BC, FAAN
Senior Vice President and Chief Nursing Officer,
University of North Carolina Hospitals
Associate Dean for UNC Health Care,
University of North Carolina at Chapel Hill School of Nursing

"*A comprehensive and readable resource for anyone starting out in clinical nursing research, whether as a direct-care clinician or graduate student. With its fresh approach and special attention to emerging topics and trends,* Anatomy of Research for Nurses *is also a unique reference for seasoned nurse researchers who facilitate studies and EBP in practice settings.*"

—Sean P. Clarke, PhD, RN, FAAN
Professor and Susan E. French Chair in Nursing Research
Innovative Practice Director,
McGill Nursing Collaborative for Education and Innovation
in Patient and Family Centered Care
Ingram School of Nursing,
Faculty of Medicine, McGill University
Editor-in-Chief, *Canadian Journal of Nursing Research*

"Anatomy of Research for Nurses *provides a clear, comprehensive, user-friendly, step-by-step approach to dissect the complicated process of nursing research for practical use by nurses in the clinical setting. The impressive credentials and rich experiences of the editors and authors, combined with their ability to make research come alive, will spark intellectual curiosity among bright professionals and have far-reaching effects for the nursing profession and patient care.*"

–Wendy C. Budin, PhD, RN-BC, FAAN
Director of Nursing Research, NYU Langone Medical Center
Adjunct Professor, New York University, College of Nursing

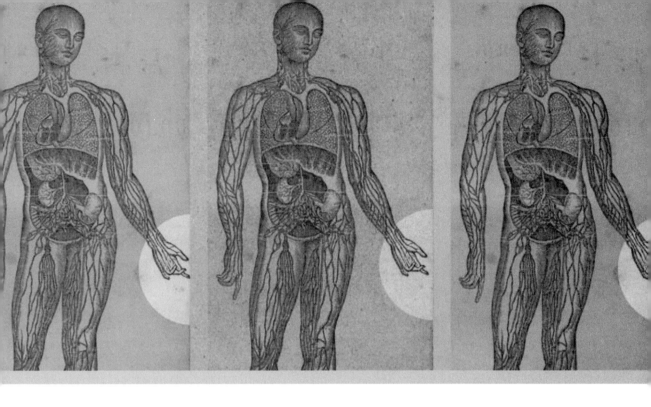

Anatomy of
RESEARCH
FOR NURSES

Christine Hedges, PhD, RN, APN

Barbara Williams, PhD, RN, APN

Sigma Theta Tau International
Honor Society of Nursing®

The Honor Society of Nursing, Sigma Theta Tau International (STTI) is a nonprofit organization whose mission is to support the learning, knowledge, and professional development of nurses committed to making a difference in health worldwide. Founded in 1922, STTI has 130,000 members in 86 countries. Members include practicing nurses, instructors, researchers, policymakers, entrepreneurs and others. STTI's 482 chapters are located at 626 institutions of higher education throughout Australia, Botswana, Brazil, Canada, Colombia, Ghana, Hong Kong, Japan, Kenya, Malawi, Mexico, the Netherlands, Pakistan, Portugal, Singapore, South Africa, South Korea, Swaziland, Sweden, Taiwan, Tanzania, United Kingdom, United States, and Wales. More information about STTI can be found online at www.nursingsociety.org.

Sigma Theta Tau International
550 West North Street
Indianapolis, IN, USA 46202

To order additional books, buy in bulk, or order for corporate use, contact Nursing Knowledge International at 888.NKI.4YOU (888.654.4968/US and Canada) or +1.317.634.8171 (outside US and Canada).

To request a review copy for course adoption, email solutions@nursingknowledge.org or call 888.NKI.4YOU (888.654.4968/US and Canada) or +1.317.634.8171 (outside US and Canada).

To request author information, or for speaker or other media requests, contact Marketing, Honor Society of Nursing, Sigma Theta Tau International at 888.634.7575 (US and Canada) or +1.317.634.8171 (outside US and Canada).

ISBN: 9781938835117
EPUB ISBN: 9781938835124
PDF ISBN: 9781938835131
MOBI ISBN: 9781938835148

Library of Congress Cataloging-in-Publication Data

Hedges, Christine, 1953- author.
  Anatomy of research for nurses / Christine Hedges, Barbara Williams.
    p. ; cm.
  Includes bibliographical references.
  ISBN 978-1-938835-11-7 (alk. paper) -- ISBN 978-1-938835-12-4 (EPUB) -- ISBN 978-1-938835-13-1 (PDF) -- ISBN 978-1-938835-14-8 (MOBI)
  I. Williams, Barbara, 1944- II. Sigma Theta Tau International, issuing body. III. Title.
  [DNLM: 1. Nursing Research. 2. Research Design. WY 20.5]
  RT81.5
  610.73072--dc23
                      2013040168

First Printing, 2014

Publisher: Renee Wilmeth

Acquisitions Editor: Emily Hatch

Editorial Coordinator: Paula Jeffers

Cover Designer: Katy Bodenmiller

Interior Design/Page Layout: Kim Scott

Principal Book Editor: Carla Hall

Development and Project Editor: Jennifer Lynn

Copy Editor: Charlotte Kughen

Proofreader: Barbara Bennett

Indexer: Joy Dean Lee

Dedication

This book is dedicated to the loving memory of my husband,
Frank Hedges, and my parents, Jim and Beth Berge,
who all believed that I could accomplish great things.
– Christine Hedges

To the memory of my parents:
my father, who taught me the "joy" of science,
and my mother, who taught me to persevere.
– Barbara Williams

Acknowledgments

As with most endeavors, this book would not have been possible without the effort and support of so many people.

We would first like to acknowledge the late Rich Hader, former Chief Nurse Executive of Meridian Health, for his vision of nursing, his inspiration, and his strong belief in the importance of research in the clinical setting.

Thank-you to Teri Wurmser, director, Meridian Health Ann May Center for Nursing and Allied Health, for her generous support throughout this project.

Thank-you to Cynthia Saver for opening the door for this opportunity and for her inspiration through *Anatomy of Writing for Publication for Nurses*.

A special thank-you to our chapter contributors both for their expertise and punctuality and for helping to create a text that is practical and useful for all nurses.

For creating illustrations for this book, thank-you to Cassie Siegel.

A heartfelt thank-you to the staff at Sigma Theta Tau International, especially Emily Hatch and Carla Hall, for their guidance, support, and patience, and to Renee Wilmeth, Jennifer Lynn, Charlotte Kughen, Barbara Bennett, Kim Scott, and Joy Dean Lee.

And last but not least, we cannot forget the appreciation for our friends, families, and coworkers for patiently supporting and putting up with us through the "birthing" of our first book!

About the Authors

Christine Hedges, PhD, RN, APN

Director, Nursing Quality and Research, UNC Health Care, Chapel Hill, NC

Christine Hedges oversees nursing quality and research initiatives at UNC Health Care. She has more than 30 years' experience in nursing and has worked in clinical practice, research, and academia. In her role as nurse scientist for the Meridian Health Ann May Center for Nursing and Allied Health, she mentored nurses who conducted research studies and evidence-based practice (EBP) projects throughout the health care system. She was also a member of the Meridian Health Institutional Review Board. Hedges has taught nursing research and EBP at Georgian Court University and William Paterson University and mentored graduate students through research and capstone projects. Hedges received her initial nursing education in Eastbourne, England; and her bachelor's and master's degrees from Columbia University, where she specialized in critical care nursing. She completed her PhD at Rutgers University where she conducted research on sleep and cognition in cardiac surgical patients. She has worked for more than 20 years as a critical care nurse and clinical nurse specialist. She is best known for her research on sleep in acute care and EBP in the hospital setting. She has authored numerous data-based articles, commentaries, and book chapters and has spoken nationally on sleep, research translation, and EBP. Hedges was the recipient of the New Jersey State Nurses Association CARES award for excellence in research in 2007; also in 2007 she was John A. Hartford Institute Geriatric Nursing Scholar; and in 2008 she was a Sigma Theta Tau International Geriatric Nursing Leadership Academy mentor. Hedges was the past research column editor and a member of the editorial board of *AACN Advanced Critical Care* and is a peer reviewer for numerous nursing journals.

Barbara Williams, PhD, RN, APN

Nurse Scientist, Meridian Health Ann May Center for Nursing and Allied Health, NJ

Barbara Williams has more than 30 years' experience in nursing as a psychiatric advanced practice nurse and more recent experience as a researcher. Her clinical experience has predominantly been in providing assessment and therapeutic interventions for patients with chronic and life-threatening illnesses, particularly on the oncology, stem cell transplant, and palliative care services in the acute care setting. In this role she has had extensive experience in working with and teaching frontline nurses. As a nurse scientist in the Meridian Health Ann May Center for Nursing and Allied Health, she conducts research and coordinates the Specialty Scholar Program in which staff nurses are mentored through research, quality improvement, and evidence-based practice (EBP) projects. Williams teaches research and EBP at William Paterson University and advises graduate students in the development and completion of research proposals. She is also a peer reviewer for *Research in Nursing and Health*.

Williams received her BSN from Seton Hall University. She received her MA in Nursing Science and her PhD in Nursing and Theory Development from New York University where in 2007 she received the Fred Schmidt Scholarship Award. She has lectured locally, regionally, and nationally on a variety of topics, including evidence-based practice, the experiences of patients with life-threatening illness, palliative care, caring, therapeutic humor, and the use of hypnosis in patient care. She has published works on the topics of patient-centered care and patients' experiences as stem cell transplant recipients.

Contributing Authors

Jane Bliss-Holtz, DNSc, RN-BC

Nurse Scientist, Meridian Health Ann May Center for Nursing and Allied Health and Co-Chair, Georgian Court-Meridian Health School of Nursing, NJ

Jane Bliss-Holtz has taught nursing research and evidence-based practice (EBP) at the undergraduate and graduate levels at the University of Pennsylvania, Rutgers College of Nursing, New Jersey City University, Thomas Edison State College, and Georgian Court University. She has published extensively and is the past editor in chief of *Issues in Comprehensive Pediatric Nursing*. She currently is employed as a nurse scientist at the Meridian Health Ann May Center for Nursing and Allied Health, which serves as a research resource for almost 2,000 nurses throughout the system. She also holds the title of co-chair of the Georgian Court-Meridian Health Baccalaureate School of Nursing. Bliss-Holtz is a graduate of University of Pennsylvania and is certified as an informatics nurse by the American Nurses Credentialing Center.

Marie Boltz, PhD, RN, GNP-BC

Assistant Professor, New York University College of Nursing, NY

Marie Boltz has extensive experience in geriatrics and gerontology as a clinician, administrator, educator, and researcher. She is an assistant professor at New York University College of Nursing, where she has served as practice director of NICHE (Nurses Improving Care for Healthsystem Elders) and is currently the associate director for research. Her research has focused on geriatric organizational models, function-focused care environments, and promoting cognitive and physical function in acutely ill, vulnerable older adults.

Catherine M. Boss, MSLS, AHIP

Coordinator, Library Services, Booker Health Sciences Library, Jersey Shore University Medical Center, NJ

Catherine M. Boss has a Master of Science degree in Library Science and is a Distinguished Member of the Academy of Health Information Professionals. Boss has been active in her profession for 40 years on the national, regional, and local levels, annually presenting papers and posters; holding positions of leadership; authoring book chapters, journal articles, and research grants; and serving as a research paper and poster judge. She has received awards for publications, leadership, presentation, and exemplary service, including being named New Jersey Health Sciences Librarian of the Year in 2002. Boss is a part-time lecturer at Rutgers University's Department of Communications and Information and serves on the school's advisory board. Currently Boss serves on the Meridian Health Institute for Evidence-Based Care Academic and Research Council as well as Jersey Shore University Medical Center's Family and Patient Education Committee and its Graduate Medical Education Committee.

Noreen B. Brennan PhD, RN

Patient Care Service Director for Medicine Surgery and Rehabilitation, Norwalk Hospital, CT

Noreen B. Brennan has been a registered professional nurse in New York for 22 years. Brennan earned her Baccalaureate of Science in Nursing from St. Francis University in Loretto, PA. She earned her Master of Arts degree in Nursing Administration and Nursing Education and her PhD from New York University. Brennan has held many nursing roles in acute care facilities, including clinical nurse for adult medical-surgical patients, clinical nurse manager, and director of nursing. In addition, Brennan served as the vice president for clinical services at Lighthouse International in New York City. Currently, Brennan is adjunct faculty at Mercy College, Dobbs Ferry, NY and New York University, NY.

Marianne Chulay, RN, PhD, FAAN

Self-employed—Consultant, Clinical Research

Marianne Chulay has more than 25 years' experience guiding, mentoring, and supporting clinician research teams in service-setting nursing organizations. In her current position as consultant in clinical research and critical care nursing, Southern Pines, NC, Chulay focuses on consultation to assist hospitals to implement and maintain an applied nursing research program that facilitates bedside clinician involvement in research projects. She is co-author of a research book, *Research Strategies for Clinicians* (Appleton & Lange, Stamford, CT, 1999) and has designed and edited several evidence-based practice resources for the American Association of Critical-Care Nurses (AACN). Chulay has more than 20 years' critical care nursing experience as a staff nurse, clinical educator, and clinical nurse specialist in a variety of critical care units in the United States and Kenya, East Africa.

Ellen Fineout-Overholt PhD, RN, FNAP, FAAN

**Dean and Professor at Groner School of Professional Studies,
Chair, Department of Nursing, East Texas Baptist University, TX**

Ellen Fineout-Overholt is a nationally recognized nursing leader, educator, and promoter of evidence-based practice (EBP) in nursing across the United States and globally. As dean of the Frank S. Groner Endowed Memorial School of Professional Studies and chair of nursing at East Texas Baptist University (ETBU), she is dedicated to building a critical mass of young leaders in nursing who will advance EBP and thereby transform health care. Fineout-Overholt was clinical professor and director for the Center for the Advancement of Evidence-based Practice at Arizona State University for seven years prior to arriving at ETBU.

Fineout-Overholt has published extensively, including serving as lead author for the group-authored "EBP Step by Step Series" in the *American Journal of Nursing*. She has been instrumental in the ongoing development of the Advancing Research & Clinical Practice through Close Collaboration (ARCC) Model and coauthored *Evidence-Based Practice in Nursing & Healthcare: A Guide to Best Practice* (2nd ed., Lippincott, Williams & Wilkins, 2011). Her newest book with Dr. Bernadette Melnyk is *Implementing Evidence-Based Practice for Nurses: Real-Life Success Stories* (Sigma Theta Tau International, 2011). Throughout her career, Fineout-Overholt has focused on developing and testing models of EBP as well as intentionally facilitating clinicians, faculty, and others to improve their craft through implementation of EBP.

James E. Galvin, MD, MPH

New York University Langone School of Medicine, NY

James E. Galvin has characterized older adults' intention to consent to dementia screening using population-based methods. He has pioneered dementia screening measures that offer quick, valid, reliable, and culturally sensitive assessments of older adults, and he has developed models characterizing the transition from healthy aging to dementia. He has directed 27 clinical trials and pioneered MRI and CSF biomarkers that identify and characterize transition to cognitive impairment related to Alzheimer's and Lewy Body dementia.

Galvin served on the Alzheimer Association National Hospital Advisory Board and led the development of a training program for hospital staff. He currently leads efforts to better understand caregiver burden, anticipatory grief, and well-being to develop interventions that benefit the patient and family alike. He directs one of the nine New York State Department of Health Alzheimer Disease Assistance Centers to provide diagnostic and social services for underserved communities. He successfully led translational research projects characterizing the clinical, cognitive, biochemical, and pathological basis of dementias resulting in 92 peer-reviewed publications and 12 book chapters in leading textbooks in geriatrics, neurology, and psychiatry.

Margo A. Halm, PhD, RN, ACNS-BC, FAHA

Director, Nursing Research, Professional Practice and Magnet, Salem Health, OR

Margo A. Halm received a PhD in Nursing from the University of Minnesota and a Master's Degree in Nursing and BSN from the University of Iowa. Currently, Halm directs the Magnet program at Salem Hospital and collaborates with interprofessional colleagues in conducting clinical research and implementing practice changes based on best available evidence. Halm also writes a regular feature column, "Clinical Evidence Review," for the *American Journal of Critical Care*; in it she unveils current evidence that supports, refutes, or sheds light on health care practices where little evidence exists. Although her main research interests focus on integrative therapies for symptom management and family caregiving after heart surgery, Halm's professional passion is igniting clinical inquiry among clinicians and assisting them to gain evidence-based practice skills to best inform their practice and affect patient outcomes.

Elizabeth Heavey, PhD, RN, CNM

Associate Professor, SUNY, Brockport, NY

Elizabeth Heavey is an associate professor and RN-BSN program director at SUNY Brockport. For 17 years she has practiced as a registered nurse and as a certified nurse-midwife with high-risk urban populations in underserved communities. She currently provides colposcopy and prenatal services in the Community Obstetrics Practice as a clinical faculty member at the University of Rochester. In addition, Heavey has a PhD in epidemiology and has completed a postdoctoral fellowship in adolescent medicine at the University of Rochester. She is the author of *Statistics for Nursing: A Practical Approach* (Jones and Bartlett, 2010). Heavey's research has focused on reproductive decision-making in high-risk adolescents, the importance of preconception care in high-risk populations, and the role of male partners in adolescent reproductive decision-making.

Shaké Ketefian, EdD, RN, FAAN
Professor Emerita (Retired), from the University of Michigan, MI

Shaké Ketefian was educated both in the United States and internationally; she has had a rich academic, scholarly, and administrative career. Throughout, she has worked extensively with U.S. and international students and has consulted with many institutions worldwide, providing curricular consultation, conducting faculty workshops, and teaching. Ketefian's research and scholarly expertise and publications have focused on research utilization, ethical issues in health care, measurement of ethical practice, research ethics, global issues in health care and knowledge development, graduate and doctoral education in the United States and worldwide. Ketefian has been editor, associate editor, editorial board member, and reviewer for many international and domestic scholarly journals. She has provided extensive service to the professional community internationally and has been recognized through many awards and honors. She is a cofounder and founding president of the International Network for Doctoral Education in Nursing. She retired from the University of Michigan School of Nursing, is Professor Emerita, and is currently serving as interim director and professor at Western Michigan University.

Richard W. Redman, PhD
Professor, University of Michigan School of Nursing, MI

Richard W. Redman is the Ada Sue Hinshaw Collegiate Chair of Nursing at the University of Michigan. He has held a number of academic administrative positions at major schools of nursing in the United States. Currently he is director of the Doctor of Nursing Practice Program. For the past six years Redman has served as chair of the Institutional Review Board for Health and Behavioral Sciences at the University of Michigan.

Kathleen Russell-Babin, PhD, RN, NEA-BC, ACNS-BC
Senior Manager, Institute for Evidence-Based Care, Meridian Health, NJ

Kathleen Russell-Babin has conducted research in nursing process, teamwork, case management, medication reconciliation, pressure ulcer attitudes, and delirium. Russell-Babin has served in leadership roles from manager to chief nursing officer. She is an American Nurses Credentialing Center (ANCC) Magnet appraiser. She has an extensive performance improvement background and has served on multidisciplinary quality improvement teams in such areas as patient satisfaction, advance directives, falls prevention, and more. In the past 3 years, Russell-Babin has led Institute for Evidence-Based Care evidence reviews on more than 30 topics. She has mentored staff nurses interested in evidence-based practice to lead teams through evidence review and implementation. She has published on topics in evidence-based care, opinion leaders, teamwork, case management, the ANCC Magnet program, and nurse retention incentives.

Claudia DiSabatino Smith, PhD, RN, NE-BC

Director of Nursing Research, St. Luke's Episcopal Hospital, Houston, TX

Claudia DiSabatino Smith is a registered nurse with 40 years' nursing experience in a variety of settings. Recently recognized with the 2012 Outstanding Alumnus Award by Mercy School of Nursing, Smith has served as the principal investigator on two research studies: one qualitative ethnographic study, from which she developed a taxonomy of clinical credibility, and one mixed methods. In addition, she has served as a coinvestigator on five nursing research studies, one of which is a $1.9 million National Institute for Occupational Safety and Health (NIOSH)–funded multisite Hospital Violence Surveillance study. In her role as the director of nursing research, she works closely with frontline nurses to develop, fund, and conduct nursing research studies and to implement best practices in the nursing care of hospitalized patients.

Karen Stonecypher, MSN, RN

Director of Education, Parkinson's Disease Research, Education and Clinical Center, Michael E. DeBakey VA Medical Center, Houston, TX

Karen Stonecypher is the former assistant clinical director for the Parkinson's Disease Research, Education and Clinical Center at the Michael E. DeBakey VA Medical Center (MEDVAMC). She received her MSN from University of Phoenix. Her clinical practice has included critical care and neurology; her research focuses on education and self-management. Stonecypher's current scholarship includes presentations and publications. She is currently pursuing her doctoral studies with a focus on nursing education from Texas Woman's University. She is a senior MEDVAMC Magnet mentor and role model for nurses implementing evidence-based projects.

Pamela Willson, PhD, RN, FNP-BC, CNE, FAANP

Director of Education, Parkinson's Disease Research, Education and Clinical Center, Michael E. DeBakey VA Medical Center, Neurology Care Line, Houston, TX

Pamela Willson is professor at the College of Nursing, Prairie View A&M University. She is former director of education for the Parkinson's Disease Research, Education and Clinical Center at the Michael E. DeBakey VA Medical Center, and faculty at Prairie View A&M University and Baylor College of Medicine, Neurology Department. She received her PhD from Texas Woman's University. She has taught advanced practice nurses for more than 25 years, and she has directed family nurse practitioner (FNP) programs and incorporated interprofessional telemedicine into the curriculum. Her clinical practice and research focuses on motor disorders, telehealth, and self-management. Current scholarship includes book chapters, presentations, and journal articles; she is co-principal investigator for an HRSA Texas Consortium Geriatric Education Center funding award in geriatric interprofessional education. She mentors nursing faculty and nurses with their theses, dissertations, and evidence-based practice projects.

Teri Wurmser, PhD, MPH, RN, NEA-BC

Director, Meridian Health Ann May Center for Nursing and Allied Health, NJ

Teri Wurmser is the director, Meridian Health Ann May Center for Nursing and Allied Health, an integrated health system in central New Jersey. The Ann May Center provides opportunities for professional growth and supports research efforts of nurses and nursing students. She recently helped to establish and is the chair of the Georgian Court-Meridian Health School of Nursing, a Bachelor in Nursing program that is a unique joint venture between a health system and a university. Wurmser graduated with a diploma in nursing from Kings County Hospital Center in Brooklyn, NY, received her BSN and PhD from Adelphi University, and MPH from Columbia University. Wurmser serves on the editorial board of *Nursing Management* and *Teaching and Learning in Nursing*, and is a ANCC Magnet program site appraiser. She has presented nationally and internationally on patient safety and enhancing the work environment for nurses.

Table of Contents

17 Research, the Internet, and Social Media: Powerful Resource or Perilous Endeavor? 277

Jane Bliss-Holtz

Foreword

As I read each chapter of *Anatomy of Research for Nurses*, I was struck by the power of an idea. I'm not talking about huge ideas, like the theory of relativity or Primary Nursing, but rather small ideas that wend their way through the mind, taking hold like a video that "goes viral" and is shared from one person to another to another in a matter of days or weeks. I've learned that small ideas often take root, eventually blossoming into robust concepts.

Many years ago, when I was senior vice president of editorial for what is now known as Nurse.com, I worked with Joan Borgatti, a nurse editor. Joan proposed the idea of critiquing an article using the analogy of anatomy. The brain represents the idea, the heart represents the flow of the article, and so on. That idea took root and blossomed in my mind, prompting me to expand on the concept and create meaningful writing workshops for nurses. Eventually, I wrote *Anatomy of Writing for Publication for Nurses* (Sigma Theta Tau International, 2010).

Now Joan's "small" idea has passed from me to research experts Christine Hedges and Barbara Williams, authors of *Anatomy of Research for Nurses*. What a perfect topic for the second book in the *Anatomy of* series. Like writing, many nurses find research daunting. Fortunately, Christine and Barbara, along with their team of top-notch contributors, walk you through challenging topics, such as analyzing data and studying special populations, with wit and wisdom.

In my role as an editorial consultant for peer-reviewed and other journals, I've worked with Christine for many years. She is an insightful peer reviewer who not only makes constructive comments that help authors improve their manuscripts, but also comments in a way that bolsters authors' confidence. Her in-depth research projects and her experience with teaching and mentoring nurses about research enable her to present information clearly and concisely in *Anatomy of Research for Nurses*.

Barbara Williams also brings the viewpoint of an experienced researcher. Her work with frontline nurses means that the information in this book has been road tested by nurses in the clinical setting who seek to do more for their patients by being savvy consumers of research and conducting their own studies, consistent with our profession's focus on evidence-based practice.

You couldn't have any better guides than Christine and Barbara on your journey to enhance your research knowledge. Their comprehensive book covers the details you need in conducting research, including settling on an idea, collecting and entering data, analyzing your findings, and disseminating results. What's most impressive is that *Anatomy of Research for Nurses* goes beyond the basics by discussing essential yet less covered topics, such as the role of social media in recruiting patients, how to keep your data secure, funding resources, legal and ethical issues, research in special populations, and how to form research teams.

Ultimately, *Anatomy of Research for Nurses* provides a valuable resource for both novice and experienced nurse researchers in all settings and for those seeking to support nurses in their efforts.

Nurses need to feel confident as consumers of research and in conducting research, whether it's a unit-based quality improvement project, an evidence-based practice project, or a multicenter randomized clinical trial. Only through research can we test out our ideas and find new ways to improve practice.

All research starts with an idea. Keep in mind that no idea is too insignificant. Your simple question as to why a certain position works better when suctioning a patient, or your innovative idea for a new strategy for teaching patients how to administer injections, or [fill in the blank!] could infect others and improve patient care.

As you read *Anatomy of Research for Nurses*, keep your tablet or pencil and paper nearby to jot down your thoughts. Complete the "Try It Now!" activities at the end of each chapter. Think about how to apply what you are learning. The ability to analyze research studies and conduct your own research is a skill you can learn, just as you learned how to start an IV or operate that new infusion pump. But like any skill, it takes knowledge and practice.

Christine and Barbara head up a team providing information and guidance that will get your neurons firing and your heart pumping with enthusiasm about research. It's up to you to transform that enthusiasm—and what you learn—into knowledge and practice. After all, some of your ideas may "go viral" too!

Cynthia Saver, RN, MS
President, CLS Development, Inc.
Columbia, MD

Introduction

"Think left and think right and think low and think high.
Oh, the thinks you can think up if only you try!"

–Dr. Seuss

Nurses on the front line have always devised innovative solutions to patient care problems, and we have not done so by haphazardly or magically pulling solutions out of a hat. We have always thought carefully about a problem, considered the science behind what we do, and then implemented and evaluated the solution.

Sound familiar? That's because it is the nursing process.

Traditionally, and for the most part, however, we have kept these solutions to ourselves— or perhaps shared them with a few colleagues. What we learned did not become part of the larger body of nursing knowledge. In other words, the solutions were not "generalizable" (you will learn more about this term as you proceed through this book).

Increasingly, however, research is the evidence upon which all health care professions are expected to base their practice (along with patient preference and clinical judgment). And although nursing research has become more common in the past few decades, the conduct of research in the clinical setting by nurses is fairly new, and we are now called upon to find innovative solutions grounded in the research process.

Nurses at every level of practice are also expected to be leaders in health care. The rich knowledge, talent, and skills possessed by nurses has not escaped the attention of national experts. In fact, in its landmark report "The Future of Nursing: Leading Change, Advancing Health," the Institute of Medicine (IOM) acknowledged that frontline nurses can play a vital role in realizing the goals of the 2010 Affordable Care Act, which is purported to be the greatest overhaul of health care since the creation of the Medicare and Medicaid programs in 1965 (IOM, 2010). Simply put, nurses are called upon to take their rightful place as leaders (along with physicians and other health care professionals) to improve the health and well-being of the nation.

And you are included in this call to action! If you previously have not been comfortable conducting research because you find it too complex, feel ill-prepared, or don't always see the relevance, this book will provide you with a practical, achievable approach to research in the clinical setting.

Research need not be daunting if you approach it as an advanced educational skill and a component of lifelong learning. Just as with any new educational skills, you don't start as an expert; instead, you learn the basics and seek out appropriate consultants and mentors to help you along the way. Do you remember when you graduated from nursing school and started your first job? Perhaps you worked on a general medical-surgical unit in an acute care hospital. You came equipped with the education and training from your initial basic licensure program. Although you were prepared and licensed to practice at an established level of competence, your nursing education didn't prepare you for everything you were likely to encounter; therefore, you were paired with a preceptor, and you quickly learned new skills to equip you to work on a specific unit or in a specific clinical setting. You started accumulating new knowledge and skills that you would need to perform at a higher level. For example, perhaps you took a course in cardiac monitoring to learn how to read and interpret ECGs or an advanced pharmacy class to learn to administer chemotherapy. After a few years, you may have decided to specialize even further by taking an advanced course in critical care, oncology, or perioperative nursing. In addition to new skills, you discovered new, diverse career opportunities. Think of acquiring beginning research skills the same way. It's an exciting opportunity!

An Anatomical Approach to Research

When you studied nursing, one of the basic courses you took was Anatomy & Physiology. You learned the following, among other things:

- How to systematically assess, physically examine, and interview a patient in order to obtain the health history, review the symptoms, examine the patient, and form a nursing diagnosis and plan of care

- How to use instruments to perform the physical examination

- How to listen to the patient's stories

- What adjustments needed to be made for special populations, such as older adults and children

You then practiced putting it all together by thinking critically. Today, you still use this approach on a daily basis with the patients in your care.

When you approach a research study systematically, whether you are conducting a study or reading one, you can think of it in terms of the anatomy; imagine the research process in a "head-to-toe" fashion (see Figure 1).

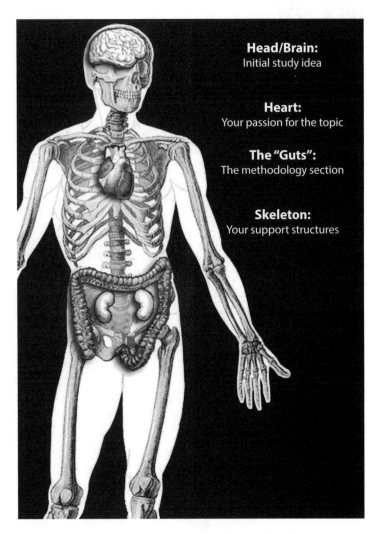

Head/Brain:
Initial study idea

Heart:
Your passion for the topic

The "Guts":
The methodology section

Skeleton:
Your support structures

Figure 1   Think about research in terms of parts of the body.

Your **head** and the **brain** represent the initial idea for the study. Where do you get great ideas for clinical questions? What is it that you think about every day that causes you to ponder and then subsequently read a research article or form a PICOT question? As your ideas become more focused, you use your brain to form research questions, hypotheses, and problem statements.

Your **heart** plays a part initially and throughout your study. Why do you want to investigate this particular phenomenon? What is the significance of this problem to nursing? As a researcher, you must have a passion for a topic! You are going to be spending time planning and executing a study, so investigate something you are interested in. Think of what you love and care about passionately. You are going to be sharing that passion with your research team.

The **"guts"**—OK, we know this isn't the real anatomical term for the abdominal organs—are the inner components, or internal "working parts." In a research study, think of these as the "Methods" (or "Methodology") section. Your design, sample, setting, and procedures are the working parts that describe how the research will be executed, and each must be carefully planned and monitored to carry out the study successfully.

The **skeleton or musculoskeletal system** of the body provides support for the entire body. In research, there are multiple support structures—for example, your carefully selected research team that represents all stakeholders required for the success of your study. Your consultants, mentors, and funding sources also provide the personal and financial support you will find invaluable for a successful outcome.

A thorough head-to-toe evaluation is not possible without your tools or physical examination equipment. Just as you rely on your stethoscope, penlight, and reflex hammer to perform your assessment in your clinical practice, you will require specialized tools to conduct research. In this book you will discover some of the important considerations of this new set of equipment.

When you studied anatomy in your nursing program, you probably learned the healthy adult anatomy first. Yet for each organ or system, you also had to learn about the differences exhibited in neonates, children, adolescents, and older adults; from there, you learned gender and cultural differences, as well as any other variations on the human anatomy. In describing how to conduct your research "head-to-toe," we will address considerations with special populations and circumstances, legal and ethical considerations, and the challenges and opportunities associated with populations, settings, technology, and the Internet in research.

Who This Book Is For

This book is intended for use primarily in the clinical setting; consequently, it differs from the more traditional research texts used in the academic setting. Although academic learning introduces nurses to the research process, the actual conduct of research can be challenging and time consuming, particularly for nurses on busy patient care units. Our aim is to provide a "practical" book for the neophyte nurse researcher on the front line. In addition, nurses transitioning from the classroom to the clinical setting can use this book. Nursing leaders, such as administrators, APNs, and nurse scientists will find this book helpful as a resource in setting up a research infrastructure in their institution or clinical setting.

How This Book Is Organized

Our book is organized in three sections.

Part I, "The Support Structure of Research," establishes the foundation for the research infrastructure in a hospital or health care setting. We also address evidence-based practice (EBP) with a frank analysis of the differences among EBP, research, and quality improvement activities, including the importance of each in knowledge generation and translation.

In Part II, "Reading and Conducting Research 'Head to Toe,'" the chapters outline the practical approach to research as we explore the steps in the research process. Analogies from clinical practice are used to illustrate challenging concepts. We conclude each chapter with a short description of how to develop and write a research proposal. We encourage nurses who are new to the research process to utilize the talents of the many consultants who are available within an organization or a partnering university. We acknowledge that not all health care settings have the same access to doctorally prepared research resources, so we provide suggestions for additional resources, such as useful websites for the new researcher. Each chapter ends with a "Try It Now!" exercise that we have frequently encountered as nurse scientists who assist clinical researchers. We highly recommend that you try the exercise at the end of each chapter to get some practice with new concepts. Leaders of newly formed nursing research committees or councils may find some of the exercises helpful in order to develop the skills of their members.

Our final section—Part III, "Important Considerations in Research"—addresses some of the important operational, legal, and ethical considerations of research, including resources on how to fund studies and work with vulnerable populations, including children, the elderly, and those persons needing additional protection in the conduct of research. These chapters provide an excellent resource for the ethical conduct of research. We conclude by addressing the exciting opportunities and challenges of conducting research in the twenty-first century as collection, storage, and transmission of data via the Internet requires all of us to learn a new set of research skills and poses a new set of questions and considerations.

Special Elements in This Book

In each chapter of *Anatomy of Research for Nurses*, you'll find these features:

- **Opening quotes:** Quotes at the start of each chapter provide pithy words of wisdom related to research.

- **Q&A sidebars:** These contain answers to some of the common questions related to the chapter's topics.

- **Try It Now!:** These exercises help you apply what you have learned.

Ready, Set, Go

Whether you are a frontline nurse (regardless of educational background), a mentor for new nurse researchers, a manager who wants to support nurse-generated research, or a CNO who wishes to develop an effective research and EBP infrastructure, we hope you will find this book a user-friendly approach to research. Let's get started!

References

Geisel, T. S. (1975). *Oh, the thinks you can think!* New York, NY: Random House.

The Support Structure of Research

I

"There is no doubt that research is a vital part of the answer to the great challenges. And excellence in research requires excellent tools. A quality research infrastructure is just as important to research as an engine is to a car."

–Morten Østergaard

Infrastructure for Nursing Research in Clinical Settings

Teri Wurmser

1

Whether you are a clinical nurse in the front lines of care or a nursing leader in your organization, it is important to begin research in a supportive environment. Nursing leadership must provide the resources needed to support nurses in research and evidence-based practice (EBP) activities. The American Nurses Credentialing Center (ANCC) Magnet® Recognition Program has been a catalyst in helping organizations develop research-rich cultures with effective infrastructures. Structures and processes that should be in place include physical and human resources, access to nurse scientists and mentors, availability of nursing research councils, financial resources, and reward and recognition mechanisms. They motivate and support direct care nurses to get involved in nursing research activities. Providing the infrastructure that supports research and innovation in an organization will provide nurses with the ability to make substantial contributions to health care and the profession. This chapter describes the elements necessary for establishing an infrastructure for nursing research in a health care organization.

WHAT YOU'LL LEARN IN THIS CHAPTER

- The infrastructure for nursing research begins with strong and committed nurse leadership.

- Nursing staff with different educational backgrounds will have various levels of expertise, and you can capitalize on this diversity.

- Personnel and structural resources are available for nursing research. Find out how to take advantage of them.

Catalysts for Nursing Research and EBP

The Institute of Medicine landmark report "The Future of Nursing: Leading Change, Advancing Health" (2010) calls for nursing professionals to take their rightful place in leading and partnering in the transformation of health care in the United States. This report states that "there will be numerous opportunities for nurses to help develop and implement care innovations" (p. 86). Nursing research provides those opportunities for nursing professionals to contribute to the science of the profession and to advance the health of patient populations. Therefore, it is imperative that nurses understand, use, and conduct research designed to have a positive effect on patient outcomes, with the ultimate goal of improving health and health care. The challenge is to create an environment within all practice settings where nurses are empowered to evaluate new knowledge and incorporate it into their clinical practice.

Q: *I am a direct care nurse, and I don't conduct research. Why do I need to get involved in research and evidence-based practice activities?*

A: As nurses, we all need to understand the role we play in generating, disseminating, and using research to improve the lives of patients. According to the International Council of Nurses, "Nurses have a professional obligation to society to provide care that is constantly reviewed, researched and validated" (ICN, 2012). Through daily interactions with patients and families, direct care nurses are in a great position to identify important clinical issues and deliver care that is grounded in new knowledge derived through research.

In addition, the ANCC Magnet Recognition Program has been a catalyst in the proliferation of research cultures across the United States. Health care practice settings that have achieved this designation or that are on the "Magnet Journey" must demonstrate that research is used in clinical decision-making and is integrated into clinical policies and procedures. Structures and processes must be in place for nurses at all levels to incorporate research findings into clinical practice and to participate in the research process. To achieve and maintain Magnet designation, organizations must be able to demonstrate that practice is based on best evidence and that nurses are empowered in their roles to use best practices to enhance the work environment and patient outcomes.

In 2007, the ANCC Magnet Recognition Program revised requirements to focus more on patient and staff outcomes (http://www.nursecredentialing.org/Magnet Model.aspx). In 2013, the *2014 Magnet Application Manual* (ANCC, 2013) further increased the emphasis on outcomes to demonstrate nursing's contribution to health care. Under the revised model, research, EBP, and quality improvement are primarily contained within the *Organizational Overview, New Knowledge, Innovations and Improvements*, and *Empirical Outcomes* components of the application. Organizations seeking Magnet designation or redesignation must provide evidence of the following:

- Nurses are knowledgeable and actively involved in the protection of human subjects.

- Resources are in place to support research and EBP.

- Nurses can articulate how they actively participate in translational activities.

- Nurses in the practice setting receive education that will help facilitate a research and EBP culture.

Evidence of an ongoing research agenda that includes studies conducted by all levels of nursing professionals is a required critical element of the application process.

The Role of Nurse Leaders

Building nursing research capacity starts with visionary leadership and organizational willingness to invest in an effective infrastructure, including investment in time, personnel, and the other resources needed to promote a culture of inquiry. Strong nurse leaders must identify barriers inherent in their own practice settings and work to creatively eliminate them (Gifford, Davies, Edwards, Griffin, & Lybanon, 2007). In tight financial times, for example, nurse leaders need to be inventive to effectively launch and sustain a culture supportive of research and innovation. For nurse executives to create an overall vision for research for their organizations, they must believe that research is vital to the nursing culture and advocate for the resources needed to realize this vision.

Barriers to Nursing Research

Many studies have identified barriers to the conduct and use of nursing research in the practice setting (Chan et al., 2011; Fink, Thompson, & Bonnes, 2005; Kelly, Turner, Gabel Speroni, McLaughlin, & Guzzetta, 2013). These barriers include the following:

- A general lack of knowledge and skills by nurses to use or conduct research
- A perceived lack of organizational and leadership support
- Time management issues
- Limited resources to conduct research
- A somewhat pervasive and general "fear" of nursing research

Organizations seeking to establish or expand nursing research capacity need to address these barriers so that nurses feel supported in their roles as consumers of and contributors to nursing research. Establishing an environment that supports the utilization and generation of research does not happen by accident; it needs to be cultivated and nurtured.

Nurse Executives

It is the role of the nurse executive to clearly articulate to the executive team, to other disciplines, to the general public, and to the nursing staff that research and EBP are essential elements of professional nursing practice. In advocating for a culture of nursing research, the nurse executive should use existing evidence that strongly ties conduct and use of research to improvements in patient outcomes and the clinical work environment. In addition, aligning research and EBP activities with the organization's strategic initiatives will help to make the case for nursing research more compelling and relevant to other members of the executive team.

Research should be clearly evident in the nursing mission and philosophy statements, and it should also be highly visible in the nursing department's model of care. An example of this is seen in the Veteran's Administration's vision and mission statements (see Figure 1.1), which highlight the belief of the importance of nursing research in the provision of quality health care. By articulating a clear mission and vision statement related to nursing research, annual research goals can more easily be established that reflect the organizational strategic initiatives, which are communicated to the nursing staff.

Improving the Health of Veterans Through Nursing Research

Vision: VA nursing research advances knowledge to promote health and excellence in healthcare for veterans and the nation.

Mission: To build capacity for high-quality research that informs evidence-based nursing practice and builds nursing science.

Source: http://www.va.gov/nursing/nursingresearch.asp

Figure 1.1   Example of nursing research vision and mission

Q: *What can I do to get direct care nurses to buy into nursing's mission and philosophy as it relates to research and EBP?*

A: The vision for research must be clearly communicated and relevant to direct care nurses in order for them to be supportive of the research mission and philosophy. Including nurses in the development and implementation of the mission and vision is vital. This can be done through the shared governance structure of the organization.

Nurse executives also can communicate expectations for nursing staff to use and participate in research through such mechanisms as nursing research councils, performance management systems, and reward and recognition programs. Also, nurse executives need to take the lead in communicating findings from nursing research to executive leadership and other members of the health care team. This would demonstrate the impact of research study outcomes that are important not only to nursing, but also to the organization. This can also set the stage for acquiring the resources necessary to maintain a robust nursing research agenda. For example, Hedges, Williams, and Tang (2013) conducted a study on the impact of national certification and clinical advancement programs on nurse engagement. Information from this study can be used to make the case for expanding support for these programs that can lead to improved patient and nurse outcomes.

Clinical Nurse Leaders

Whereas the nurse executive provides the vision for research within an organization, nurse leaders at all levels must assure that this vision is translated into action at the point of care. The challenge of balancing staff development and participation in the research process with assuring provision of quality direct patient care can be daunting for frontline nurse managers. Frontline nurse leaders need to understand that nursing research can help them to achieve their unit goals and can have a positive impact on unit outcomes. Leaders can support direct care nurses by encouraging clinical questioning, by providing time and resources for their staff to participate in research and EBP, and by highlighting and recognizing staff-led activities to the rest of the staff and the organization.

An important step in assisting frontline nurse leaders in their own beliefs of the efficacy of fostering nursing research activities would be to identify successful examples of the use of research evidence and resultant improved clinical outcomes. Additionally, understanding of the barriers for staff participation in nursing research is important in assisting nurse leaders to identify these barriers in their own environments and to develop action plans. Frontline nurse leaders should consider a multifaceted approach to eliminating these barriers, including supporting education, providing mentoring, and offering release time to attend meetings and conduct research (Fink, Thompson, & Bonnes, 2005).

Preparation and Expectations of the Nursing Staff

Many nurses feel ill-prepared to evaluate and utilize research findings or to independently conduct research, so it is important to have a grasp of what can reasonably be expected of frontline staff nurses within an organization. In its 2006 *Position Paper on Nursing Research,* the American Association of Colleges of Nursing (AACN) outlined the expected research competencies of graduates from all levels of nursing education programs. According to this AACN expert panel, nurses at the bachelor's level should be prepared to evaluate and apply research findings within the practice setting, to assist in the development of research questions, and to serve on research teams. Thus, dependent solely on educational level, staff nurses may not necessarily have the skill set to develop a research protocol or conduct research on their own.

Q: *I am a bachelor's prepared nurse working in a university-affiliated health care organization. I would like to conduct a research study on my unit, but do not know how to get started. Help!*

A: If your organization has a medical library, start there. Work with the medical librarian to conduct a literature search on your topic. Collect and start reviewing the literature on your area of interest. If your organization has a research committee or council, start attending meetings to learn what others are doing. You can discuss your ideas and get feedback from your peers on the project you would like to conduct. Also, consider working with a team. Ask yourself, "Who else might be interested in my research question?" If there is a nurse scientist or research consultant in your organization, schedule a meeting or look for a mentor with research experience who can help you through the steps of the research process.

Research competency increases with advanced degree preparation, and nurses with the terminal research degree are those who are most able to fully conduct research. Newer roles such as the clinical nurse leader (CNL) and the doctor of nursing practice (DNP) are knowledgeable in aspects of the cycle of integration of evidence into practice, and the skills that they bring are especially useful in translational activities that support a culture of research and EBP in the practice setting.

To establish a vibrant and effective nursing research culture, an organization should capitalize on the education and experience of nurses from a variety of educational backgrounds by using these nurses in different capacities. Table 1.1 is a summary of the expected skill set for nursing research based on education level (AACN, 2006).

Table 1.1   Levels of Education and Expectations for Research Competencies

Education Level	Expectations
Bachelor's Degree in Nursing	Understand the research process and elements of EBP at the basic level
	Understand and apply research findings from nursing and other disciplines in clinical practice
	Work with others to identify potential research questions
	Collaborate on research teams
Master's Degree in Nursing	Evaluate research findings
	Develop and implement EBP guidelines
	Form and lead interprofessional teams
	Identify issues that require study
	Collaborate with scientists in the conduct of research

continues

Table 1.1   Levels of Education and Expectations for Research Competencies *continued*

Education Level	Expectations
Clinical Nurse Leader (CNL)	Evaluate evidence for practice
	Implement EBP
	Use quality improvement strategies to affect improved outcomes at the microsystem level
	Identify clinical problem areas
	Participate in the implementation of clinical research.
Doctor of Nursing Practice (DNP)	Translate research into practice
	Evaluate evidence
	Apply research in decision-making
	Implement clinical innovations and best evidence to change practice
Research Doctorate (PhD, DNSc)	Conduct independent research for the purpose of extending knowledge
	Plan and execute an independent program of research
	Involve and mentor others (i.e., students, clinicians, and other researchers) in scholarly activities and research

Personnel Resources for Nursing Research

Having individuals familiar with the research and EBP process is an essential ingredient for creating a research rich culture. Internal and/or external "experts" with the right skill sets must be available to guide the novice researcher in the right direction. These experts bring the knowledge, leadership, talent, and passion to move research agendas forward. Hiring nurses with extensive research and EBP skills or growing your own are ways to increase availability of internal experts. Finding external experts to serve as consultants and provide the needed expertise to support an organization's research mission is yet another way to accomplish this goal.

Internal Research Consultants

As most nursing staff do not feel educationally or experientially prepared for research activities, the availability of key personnel who possess research skills and experience can help launch and sustain research activities within the organization. Initiation of the position of a doctorally prepared nurse scientist within an organization can assure the presence of an internal consultant who can assist in building and maintaining an effective nursing research infrastructure. Jamerson and Vermeersch (2012) noted that a full-time position is preferred because full-time nurse scientists better understand the organization's culture, have a stronger commitment to the organization, and have a firmer grasp of the needs and available resources of the organization. Additionally, having a full-time nurse scientist provides the opportunity to focus attention on building nursing research resources and can lead to the establishment of a center for nursing research within an organization.

Q: *What benefits would a center for nursing research bring to an organization and its nurses?*

A: A center for nursing research can consolidate many of the resources needed to promote and sustain a research rich culture and can lead to tangible increases in participation in all levels of research. By investing in a center for nursing research, the foundation for meeting the research and EBP criteria for Magnet designation can be established.

External Research Consultants

For many nursing departments, hiring a doctorally prepared nurse scientist may not be feasible. Alternatives include hiring external research consultants on an ongoing basis or partnering with educational institutions to form joint appointments with faculty.

The Role of the Research Consultant

Whether a full-time nurse scientist, a part-time research consultant, or a faculty collaborator, the role of the doctorally prepared nursing research consultant includes:

- Attending research committee meetings

- Working with nursing staff on searching and critiquing research literature

- Developing and conducting research studies

- Assisting staff in preparing abstracts for podium or poster presentations and research publications

If the nursing research consultant has an established program of research, then nursing staff can participate as members of the research team, which enables them to learn the research process.

The Role of Research Mentors

Another strategy that has been successful in promoting a research culture is the use of research mentors. Mentors are commonly used in university settings to assist novice researchers, who benefit from the expertise of seasoned research scholars (Ulrich & Grady, 2003; Byrne & Keefe, 2002; AACN, 2006). Using academia as a model, mentors can be very effective in the practice setting as well. Unlike consultants, who have limited time and investment in the projects in which they consult, research mentors take more of an active role and guide novice nurse researchers through the entire research process—from idea generation to dissemination of the findings.

 Are research mentors really that important?

 The availability of research mentors was cited as the top *facilitator* of nursing research in both Magnet and non-Magnet hospitals, whereas lack of mentors was the most frequently cited *barrier* to research in non-Magnet hospitals (Kelly, Turner, Gabel Speroni, McLaughlin, & Guzzetta, 2013).

An advantage to a research mentorship program is that staff who have been successfully mentored can serve as research mentors to the next generation of nursing staff. These research mentors can offer advice and counsel on a "been there, done that" basis as well as serve as cheerleaders for project progress. Providing training and other resources for mentors (such as "time back" for facilitating) can help to promote a successful mentorship relationship and program (Byrne & Keefe, 2002).

Structural Resources for Nursing Research

In addition to the human capital, other elements need to be in place to support a research infrastructure. These structural resources include availability of library and online literature search resources, access to funds for research purposes, processes to protect human subjects in the conduct of research, and nursing committees/councils and journal clubs.

Onsite and Online Literature Search Resources

A basic ingredient of an effective research infrastructure is the availability of library and literature search resources. An onsite library with dedicated and highly skilled medical librarians can provide invaluable support to both novice and experienced researchers. Enlisting the help of medical librarians who provide hands-on education at convenient times for staff nurses can help make searching the literature a less onerous task. Onsite and online access to databases and full text journals also is desirable. (Chapter 6 provides a listing of free online resources.)

In addition to online search engines, a dedicated nursing research web page on the institution's website can be very effective in promoting a research culture. The dedicated site might include any or all of the following:

- Meeting minutes for the nursing research council
- Research and EBP toolkits
- Online educational offerings, including webinars and video recordings of live conferences
- Workshops
- Newsletters
- Research blogs

A webmaster should be responsible for maintaining and updating the website on a regular basis.

Financial Resources

Obviously, there are costs associated with implementing an effective research infrastructure. Nursing leaders need to consider these costs when advocating for resources to support research in the clinical setting. In addition to personnel costs for dedicated nurse scientists, other costs might include:

- Expenses associated with full text online databases and journals
- Statistical software for analyzing research results
- Biostatistician support
- Data entry costs

- Printing costs

- Survey-associated expenses (such as stamps or a subscription to an online survey tool)

- Dissemination expenses (including poster development, conference registration, and travel expenses)

Speaker costs for research conferences and workshops can also be a significant expense; however, they can yield a high return on investment in getting nurses engaged and excited about research.

Processes to Protect Human Subjects

An important element in the establishment of a research infrastructure is the availability of processes and procedures for the protection of human subjects in research. All nurses within an organization, whether they plan to conduct a study or not, need to have a basic understanding of the role of the Institutional Review Board (IRB) in the protection of human subjects. As primary patient advocates, nurses have an ethical responsibility to assure that the rights of research participants are respected and upheld, which requires knowledge of the regulations and policies that govern ethical research. Furthermore, nurse leaders should assure that there is nursing representation in the voting membership of the IRB. You can find more information on ethics in research at Bioethics Resources on the Web (http://bioethics.od.nih.gov) and in Chapter 14 of this book.

Nursing Research Councils/Committees

A nursing research council or committee is an important element of the infrastructure for nursing research. The goal of a research council is to support and encourage nursing staff involvement in research activities (Fowler, Leaton, Baxter, McTigue, & Snook, 2008).

Research councils can be part of the shared governance structure within the organization, ultimately communicating to the overall nursing decision-making body. Ideally, members of a research council include at least one volunteer member from each of the units/departments within the organization as well as nurses experienced in reading and translating research, such as advanced practice nurses (APNs). The functions of nursing research councils include the following:

- Staff education

- Facilitation of the organization's research agenda

- Provision of opportunities to disseminate research results both internally and externally

- Promotion of utilization of research findings

As the council membership gains expertise in the research process, members can offer assistance to other nursing staff who are interested in conducting their own studies. Additionally, the council may undertake small-scale research projects as a group. In some organizations, these councils provide peer review for nursing research studies to assure scientific merit and integrity, serving as a review process prior to IRB submission.

A nursing research council can be started by inviting interested nurses to attend an inaugural meeting. APNs and nurse educators should be included, as they have some knowledge of the research process from their graduate education; they can serve as effective champions for nursing research to a variety of constituencies as well as provide leadership to help meet council goals and objectives. Additionally, APNs work with challenging patient populations that offer the potential to generate relevant research questions. Support of unit managers also should be solicited, as they can identify potential council members from their units. Placing an announcement of the first research council meeting on the agenda of the organization's central nursing practice council also can assist in gaining members.

The first research council meeting should be held on a day and time that is most convenient for interested staff to attend, and the agenda should be kept manageable; an hour of a timed agenda would be ideal, with time for introductions and "ice-breaking" activities. Agendas for subsequent meetings might include the development of a mission statement and bylaws, establishment of regular meeting dates and times, and articulation of a set of short- and long-term goals. Council goals may include developing a process for assessing needs and barriers to research for the nursing staff and developing a basic educational plan for both the committee and for the rest of the organization. At early meetings, the council might brainstorm to identify some of the research resources that are available within the organization and also identify some activities to generate interest in nursing research among the nursing staff.

Q: *What kinds of activities will generate interest in nursing research?*

A: Spreading the word about the importance of nursing research among stakeholders can be accomplished in many ways.

You can generate interest by initiating journal clubs where staff collaborate on the review of research studies that might be relevant to practice. Consider inviting staff who are not members to a nursing research council meeting and buddy them with members. Another strategy is to host a "Research and EBP" week or month where studies are presented either in poster or podium presentations. Many organizations have research newsletters or publications. Make sure that nursing studies are featured if the publication is not nursing specific. However you decide to highlight nursing research activities, be sure to be creative in your approach.

As the council develops, functions may evolve to a more active role in supporting, reviewing, and generating nursing research, in dissemination activities, and in review of proposed research projects for scientific merit prior to IRB review. An example of review criteria is presented in Figure 1.2.

Other functions of mature nursing research councils may include planning educational programs, such as facility-wide poster presentations, nursing grand rounds, and full-scale conferences that highlight nursing research and EBP projects. Dependent on an organizational needs assessment, programs may include such topics as the steps in the research process, ethical considerations in conducting research, how to develop poster and PowerPoint nursing research presentations, and writing for publication. Bringing in nationally recognized speakers to present their research at an annual research day can create excitement and be a motivating force for staff.

Journal Clubs

Journal clubs can be a good means for nurses unfamiliar with research to gain experience in reading and critiquing research articles and to stay abreast of current research in the field (Kleinpell, 2002; Kirchoff & Beck, 1995). Journal clubs have been used to promote nursing research awareness (Luby, Riley, & Towne, 2006) and as a means of facilitating EBP (Dyckoff, Manela, & Valente, 2004; Kartes & Kamel, 2003; Vratny & Shriver, 2007). As an easily implemented and cost-effective strategy, journal clubs have the potential to change nurses' attitudes toward research, to reduce perceived barriers to research utilization in nursing practice (O'Nan, 2011), and to promote research use on individual units and in specialty areas.

Example of Research Protocol Review Criteria (Meridian Health)			
Title	Acceptable	Not Acceptable	Accepted With Revision
1. Topic Topic is interesting, timely, and clinically applicable.			
2. Title page			
3. Abstract Abstract is a clear representation of the study.			
4. Research question/problem statement/hypothesis Central concepts or variables are clearly identified.			
5. Definition of terms All terms are clearly defined.			
6. Significance to nursing			
7. Review of the literature Relevant and recent literature is clearly presented.			
8. Subjects (sample) Type of sampling, sample size, and sample characteristics are clearly described.			
9. Instruments Instruments are clearly described, reliable, and valid.			
10. Design Design is clearly described and appropriate.			
11. Proposed data analysis Data analysis is clearly described and appropriate.			
12. Ethical considerations and consent form Ethical considerations are clearly described and appropriate.			
13. References			
14. Grammar and composition clear and appropriate			

_____ Recommend for approval

_____ Recommend for approval with minor revisions

_____ Recommend for approval with major revisions

Figure 1.2   Example of research protocol review criteria (Meridian Health)

Planning a Journal Club

The Oncology Nursing Society has developed a useful toolkit that is available on the Web to help you get started in planning a journal club at your institution (http://www.ons.org/publications/media/ons/docs/publications/ journalclubtoolkit.pdf).

Virtual journal clubs are becoming more and more popular as a method of overcoming the barrier of lack of time to attend meetings (Lehna, Berger, Truman, Goldman, & Topp, 2010; Berger, Hardin, & Topp, 2011). An example of this is found at Baptist Health Care System in Florida, which has implemented a "Traveling Journal Club." Nurses can access research articles for review on their intranet and respond to others' comments in an online blog.

Mentored Research Programs for Frontline Nursing Staff

Many organizations with commitment to promoting nursing research have established mentoring programs to support frontline nursing staff through the steps of a research project. These programs are generally very structured, with a standardized curriculum and regularly scheduled meetings over the course of 1 to 2 years. After the research mentorship is completed, opportunities for internal dissemination of research results are built into the program so that novice nurse researchers have the opportunity to present in front of an audience.

Meridian Health (MH), a health care system in central New Jersey, has established a Specialty Scholar Program as part of its CARE (Clinical Advancement and Recognition of Excellence) program. Nurses who agree to participate in this program can advance to the highest level of CARE and receive an increase in hourly salary after completing the application and education. Specialty scholars in the program must complete one project in the areas of research, EBP, or quality. Nurses attend a 3-day educational program taught by a faculty of nurse scientists and other experts (see Figure 1.3 for an example of the Specialty Scholar curriculum outline) and are assigned a mentor. At the completion of their projects, specialty scholars are required to present their outcomes during at least one of several scheduled conferences, including the annual MH Research Day, the annual Nursing Research and EBP conference, or the annual MH Geriatric NICHE (Nurses Improving Care for Health System Elders) Conference.

Meridian Health Clinical Specialty Scholar Curriculum	
Day	**Topic**
Day 1	Overview of Curriculum and the Specialty Scholar Program Benchmarking Basics Introduction to Research and Protection of Human Subjects Introduction to Evidence-Based Practice Resources for Specialty Scholars Topic Development Expectations of Specialty Scholar Communications
Day 2	Recap of Day 1 Deming's Methodology for Process Improvement: Plan Do Check Act
Day 3	Overview of Quality, EBP or Research Scholar (Three tracks, participant selects track according to clinical question)

Figure 1.3   Meridian Health Clinical Specialty Scholar Curriculum

This program has become an effective way to engage nursing staff in projects that improve outcomes and encourage nurses at all levels to participate in knowledge translation activities. The program also highlights nursing research and EBP efforts throughout the organization and provides a forum to acknowledge and recognize nursing's contribution to science and innovation.

Reward and Recognition

Reward and recognition is an important component of a research infrastructure. Nursing research is a labor-intensive activity that requires commitment and time above and beyond what is usually required of the practicing nurse. It is important to include mechanisms to reward and recognize nurses who take the initiative to become involved in nursing research, as their efforts have the potential to improve patient care. Nurses who participate in research activities can be recognized in internal organizational publications, in nursing research newsletters, and during staff and research council meetings.

In addition, funds can be provided for nurses to attend research conferences to learn more about the field or to present the results of their projects. Financial and nonfinancial incentives can be excellent motivators for nurses to become actively involved. Nonfinancial motivators might include time off to attend meetings and protected time to conduct research activities. Including research activities in the clinical recognition program (clinical ladder) also can be used as a financial incentive. Availability of competitive small grants within the institution to conduct research can serve as an incentive as well.

Funding Nursing Research

The need for financial resources to support nursing research was mentioned earlier in this chapter. Although operating budgets for nursing research and EBP activities are important, there are other sources of funding that can be tapped to support and propel nursing research within an organization. Opportunities for funding to support practice and research initiatives are available for nurses who seek them out (Wurmser & Hedges, 2009). Searching the Internet and working with the organization's grants department are two good methods to find funding sources to support your special projects and full-scale research studies. (You can learn more about funding in Chapter 16 of this book.)

Try It Now!

Explore websites of Magnet Organizations (see http://www.nursecredentialing.org/FindaMagnetHospital.aspx to find a list of Magnet hospitals) to see how nursing research and evidence-based practice are highlighted. Compare these websites to your organization's website. How does your organization compare? What would you like to see changed? Who would you speak to about making these changes to highlight nursing research at your institution?

References

American Association of Colleges of Nursing. (2006). *Position Paper on Nursing Research.* Retrieved from http://www.aacn.nche.edu/publications/position/nursing-research

American Nurses Credentialing Center. (2013). *2014 Magnet Application Manual.* Silver Springs, MD: Author.

Berger, J., Hardin, H. K., & Topp, R. (2011). Implementing a virtual journal club in a clinical nursing setting. *Journal of Nurses in Staff Development, 27*(3), 116–120. doi 10.1097NND.0b013e318217b3bc

Byrne, M., & Keefe, M. (2002). Building research competence in nursing through mentoring. *Journal of Nursing Scholarship, 34*(4), 391–396.

Chan, G. K., Barnason, S., Dakin, C. L., Gillespie, G., Kamienski, M. C., Stapleton, S., … Li, S. (2011). Barriers and perceived needs for understanding and using research among emergency nurses. *Journal of Emergency Nursing, 37*(1), 24–31. doi:101016/j.jen.2009.11.016

Dyckoff, D., Manela, J., & Valente, S. (2004). Improving practice with a journal club. *Nursing, 34*(7), 29.

Fink, R., Thompson, C. J., & Bonnes, D. (2005). Overcoming barriers and promoting the use of research in practice. *Journal of Nursing Administration, 35*(3), 121–129.

Fowler, S., Leaton, M. B., Baxter, T., McTigue, T., & Snook, N. (2008). Evolution of nursing research committees. *Journal of Neuroscience Nursing, 40*(1), 60–63.

Gifford, W., Davies, B., Edwards, N., Griffin, P., & Lybanon, V. (2007). Managerial leadership for nurses' use of research evidence: An integrative review of the literature. *Worldviews on Evidence Based Nursing, 4*(3), 126–145.

Hedges, C., Williams, B. J., & Tang, C. (2013). Conference proceedings: RCN 2013 Annual International Research Conference, Belfast. Retrieved from http://www.rcn.org.uk/development/researchanddevelopment/rs/2013_-_annual_conference/posters_2013

Institute of Medicine. (2010). The future of nursing: Leading change, advancing health. Retrieved from http://books.nap.edu/openbook.php?record_id_12956&page=R1

International Council of Nurses. (2012). Closing the gap: From evidence to action. ICN: Geneva, Switerland. Retrieved from http://www.icn.ch/images/stories/documents/publications/ind/indkit2012.pdf

Jamerson, P. A., & Vermeersch, P. (2012). The role of the nurse research facilitator in building research capacity in the clinical setting. *Journal of Nursing Administration, 42*(1), 21–28. doi: 10.1097/NNA.0b013e31823c180e

Kartes, S., & Kamel, H. K. (2003). Geriatric journal club for nursing: A forum to enhance evidence-based nursing care in long-term settings. *Journal of the American Medical Directors Association, 4*(5), 264–267.

Kelly, K. P., Turner, A., Gabel Speroni, K., McLaughlin, M. K., & Guzzetta, C. (2013). National survey of hospital nursing research, part 2: Facilitators and hindrances. *Journal of Nursing Administration, 43*(1), 18–23.

Kirchoff, K. T., & Beck, S. L. (1995). Using the journal club as a component of the research utilization process. *Heart & Lung, 24*, 246–250.

Kleinpell, R. (2002). Rediscovering the value of the journal club. *American Journal of Critical Care, 11*(5), 412–414.

Lehna, C., Berger, J., Truman, A., Goldman, M., & Topp, R. (2010) Virtual journal club connects evidence to practice: An analysis of participant responses. *Journal of Nursing Administration, 40*(12), 522–528. doi: 10.1097/NNA.0b013e318fc19c0

Luby, M., Riley, J., & Towne, G. (2006). Nursing research journal clubs: Bridging the gap between practice and research. *Medsurg Nursing, 15*, 100–102.

O'Nan, C. (2011). The effect of a journal club on perceived barriers to utilization of nursing research in a practice setting. *Journal for Nurses in Staff Development, 27*(4), 160–164.

Ulrich, C., & Grady, C. (2003). Research mentors: An understated value. *Nursing Research, 52*(3), 139.

United States Department of Veteran Affairs. (nd). VA Nurses research and vision statements. Retrieved from http://www.va.gov/nursing/nursingresearch.asp

Vratny, A., & Shriver, D. (2007). A conceptual model for growing evidence-based practice. *Nursing Administration Quarterly, 31*(2), 162–170.

Wurmser, T., & Hedges, C. (2009). A primer for successful grant writing. *Advanced Critical Care, 26*(1), 102–107.

EBP, QI, and Research: Strange Bedfellows or Kindred Spirits?

2

Ellen Fineout-Overholt

WHAT YOU'LL LEARN IN THIS CHAPTER

- EBP, QI, and research have different purposes.

- EBP, QI, and research have different processes.

- Worldviews influence clinical decision-making.

- EBP, QI, and research can assist clinicians in achieving best practice.

Another name for kindred spirit could be soul mate. There is an integration or interwoven aspect to this kind of relationship that transcends any differences. In Lucy Maude Montgomery's book *Anne of Green Gables* (1908), the main character, Anne, is an orphan whose primary desire is to be loved. She craves a true kindred spirit with whom she can share her perceptions, experiences, adventures and failures…knowing that her kindred spirit friend will share all of these with authenticity.

Strange bedfellows, on the other hand, are not kindred spirits. Rather, they are thrown into association through some untoward circumstance. They do not necessarily share common interests or goals. The entire premise of the 1970s U.S. television show *The Odd Couple* (Marshall, 1970–1975) was the mismatch between two gentlemen who had different goals, processes (habits), and purposes (goals in life) but were thrown together out of necessity.

In health care, there seem to be different perspectives about how evidence-based practice (EBP), quality improvement (QI), and research fit within our approach to care. This chapter focuses on clarifying this confusion and helping clinicians consider their perspective and determine how to best utilize these processes to benefit their practice and the patients for whom they care. When you have completed reading this chapter, it is hoped that you will be decidedly confident about whether EBP, QI, and research are kindred spirits or strange bedfellows.

Worldviews Matter: Why and How Decisions Are Made

A worldview is how you approach life—in the case of a nurse, it is how you approach caring for your patients. The decisions you make on a daily basis are grounded in your worldview. Your chosen worldview impacts your priorities, your choices, how you use your resources, and how you spend your money.

Specific worldviews lead to the various understandings of how clinicians care for patients. For example, a person with a biomedical worldview focuses on the symptoms, illness, and treatment, whereas a person with a holistic worldview has an integrated focus on the whole person. Clinicians will make different decisions based on which worldview is driving them. Biomedical clinicians will treat to mitigate symptoms, using such interventions as medicines and surgical interventions, for example, whereas clinicians with a holistic worldview will consider these options as well as what the whole person needs to achieve optimal health, including what may be considered alternative interventions, such as counseling, massage, aromatherapy, imagery, and exercise.

Each worldview has facilitating factors that help it thrive and barriers that keep it from being adopted as the overall worldview of health care. Given that nurses are the people who drive decisions at the bedside and beyond through their observations, questions, and ideas (Raines, 2012), their worldviews matter and will influence patient and provider outcomes.

Definitions are basic to understanding different worldviews, as are the questions they answer (see Table 2.1).

Table 2.1 Questions Answered by Different Worldviews

Question for EBP	What is the most reliable approach for achieving the best outcomes for our patients?
Question for QI	How are the things working that we are currently using to manage our patients?
Question for Research	Where are the gaps in what we know about health/patient care? For example, gaps about (1) the relationship between treatment options and outcomes [quantitative approach]; (2) how individuals or groups experience health care and/or disease [qualitative approach]; (3) the implications and nuances of intervention delivery methods [translational research]; (4) how to effectively change systems/processes [health services research; implementation science]?

Evidence-Based Practice

Sackett, Strauss, Richardson, Rosenberg, and Haynes (2000) defined evidence-based practice (EBP) as the conscientious use of current best evidence in making decisions about patient care. The definition of EBP has evolved in scope to refer to a lifelong problem-solving approach to clinical decision-making that incorporates the following (Melnyk & Fineout-Overholt, 2011):

1. A systematic search for and critical appraisal and synthesis of the most relevant and best research (i.e., external evidence) to answer a burning clinical question

2. One's own clinical expertise, which includes internal evidence generated from outcomes management or quality improvement projects, a thorough patient assessment, and evaluation and use of available resources necessary to achieve desired patient outcomes

3. Patient values and preferences

There is no specific formula for combining these aspects of the EBP worldview; however, all should be present when making clinical decisions.

Every clinical encounter offers the opportunity to individually care for a particular patient in such a way that brings about the best outcome for that patient. For example, evidence from research might support the efficacy of one anticoagulant medication over another in preventing deep vein thrombosis in at-risk patients. However, if a patient experiences adverse side effects from the preferred medication and refuses to take it, patient preference outweighs the evidence from research. As a result, the health care provider should choose an alternative anticoagulant to administer to the patient.

Evidence-Based Practice Paradigm Conceptual Framework

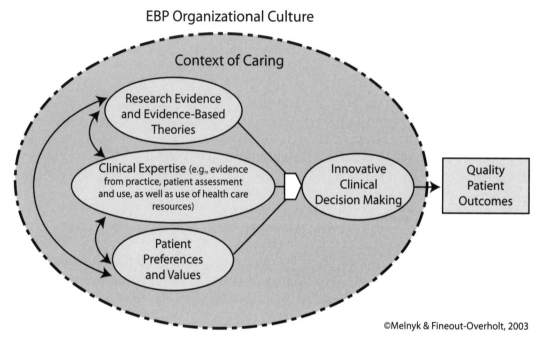

Figure 2.1   The EBP paradigm

In other situations, the internal evidence, such as data from patient assessment, hospital records, quality improvement projects, or available resources drives the decision that will achieve the outcome (Melnyk & Fineout-Overholt, 2011). EBP results in the best clinical decisions and patient outcomes when it is delivered in a context of caring and is supported by an organizational culture for EBP, as shown in Figure 2.1 (Melnyk & Fineout-Overholt, 2003).

Quality Improvement

Quality improvement (QI) is an internal process by which processes and outcomes of practice are evaluated for quick intervention in an organization. QI also has been referred to as *performance improvement (PI)*. There are various models for QI; however, most started with the Deming Model (1982) and incorporate the plan, do, study (sometimes called *check*), act (PDSA) cycle. (Note: Study in this case does not mean conduct a methodological study; rather, it means observe what has happened, or *check* what has happened.) Deming described this QI cycle as iterative, meaning that the phases of the cycle influence each other and how the cycle is working. More recent renditions of this approach that are primarily focused on processes include Six Sigma's define, measure, analyze, improve, control (DMAIC) and Lean methodologies (Varkey & Kollengode, 2011).

Although these approaches allow for trialing or testing of processes, it is important to note that trialing an intervention without adequate external evidence to support the reliability of the intervention and expected outcome may lead to less than optimal outcomes (Cepero, 2011). Despite that, the PDSA approach is thought to have been born out of the scientific method (Lamber & Shearer, 2010); use of this approach to problem-solve does not guarantee that generalizable information will be produced. That being said, it is important to recognize that QI provides wonderful opportunities to consider what clinical issues are ripe for research.

In QI, there is a need to collect preliminary data before moving into the planning phase of PDSA. An approach called *FOCUS PDSA* (see Figure 2.2) offers opportunity for the QI

Quality Improvement Cycle (FOCUS-PDSA)	
Find...	a process to improve
Organize...	the team
Clarify...	current knowledge about the process
Understand...	what is creating the differences that brought the issue to your attention
Select...	processes, benchmarks, and QI tools that will improve the outcomes
Plan...	what will happen when you implement the process
Do...	what you plan and collect data on what happened
Study...	analyze how well the plan brought about the expected results and lessons learned
Act/Adjust...	based on the study phase, adjust next steps and revise plan
FOCUS-PDSA cycle repeats	

Figure 2.2   The quality improvement cycle

team to gather and assess more data on the front end of the process; however, evidence and research are not necessarily a part of these data. QI offers insight into efficiencies of processes; however, as a method of addressing change, QI does not consistently consider the role of external evidence (i.e., research), which distinguishes it from EBP.

Research

Research is defined as the systematic discovery or validation of generalizable knowledge (Polit & Beck, 2011). The knowledge must be usable beyond those who generated it—this is what makes it "generalizable." Research has long been the mainstay of many disciplines that established themselves as professions, such as nursing, medicine, and bench sciences. There are different approaches to how this worldview of new knowledge generation operates in everyday life, with the quantitative and qualitative approaches being the most common. The *quantitative approach* encompasses counting and measuring outcomes, such as how many patients have deep vein thrombosis. *Qualitative approaches* encompass the experience of the person with the deep vein thrombosis and describe what contributes to that experience (context). Research offers new information for clinicians to use in practice. This worldview holds that research is the pinnacle of the profession and the conduct of research is paramount.

Integration of Worldviews for Best Practice

The EBP, QI, and research worldviews are not mutually exclusive; rather, they are integrated into a best practice approach to health care that will consistently deliver outcomes for patients and the organization/system (Shirey et al., 2011). There is overlap in the processes of each worldview that is critical to understanding how to best use them to achieve the goal of best practice. Consider further that the primary process in health care to achieve best outcomes is the EBP process, into which the QI and research processes dovetail.

It is helpful to think of these relationships as an umbrella: EBP is the overarching umbrella; research serves as the handle and tube of the umbrella that supports EBP; and QI is the spine-like stretchers of the umbrella itself (see Figure 2.3). The umbrella function can be assessed by how well the stretchers hold up to the weather. Sometimes there is a little droop on one side because that stretcher is slightly bent (e.g., monitored data indicate a need to examine processes), but the umbrella still functions; however, sometimes, the stretcher breaks, and at that time there is need for major repair (e.g., critical incident occurs; new process developed). The handle and tube are critical to the function of the umbrella. If they are too small (e.g., insufficient evidence), the umbrella doesn't stand up to the elements. If they are faulty (i.e., poorly conducted research), the umbrella may fail. However, with a sturdy, functional handle and tube, the umbrella functions well in all weather—that is, it is reliable.

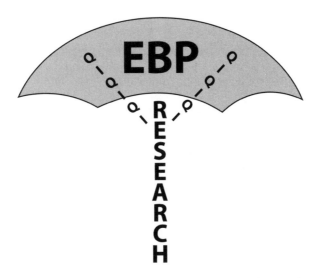

Figure 2.3   The relationship between EBP, QI, and research

Although the umbrella analogy may be imperfect, it is helpful to understanding the integration of EBP, QI, and research. To further help in understanding this integration, let us consider keywords that may serve as a beginning understanding of these three worldviews:

- EBP *translates* that best available evidence into clinical practice to achieve the best quality of care and patient outcomes.

- QI *monitors* ongoing practice.

- Research *generates* new knowledge for use in practice when evidence does not exist.

> **Q:** *Nurses on our unit reported that they had data from our risk management system that indicated that there was a major issue on our unit with falls. The staff got together and decided to implement a color-coded arm band according to the risk of the patient. What is this: EBP, QI, or research?*
>
> **A:** QI. This is ongoing monitoring of practice. The decision to use color-coded armbands was because someone had gone to a conference and heard it worked. The team did not formulate a PICOT question or do a search to find best evidence. They conducted a small test of change using PDSA to see if their idea worked.

Q: *A clinical nurse specialist (CNS), nurse practitioner, staff nurse, and nurse educator were discussing the literature on using cola to unclog NG (nasogastric) tubes. The CNS is PhD prepared and indicated to the group that there is not sufficiently reliable evidence to support this process. She suggested that they need to determine reliably whether or not cola is an effective treatment for clogged NG tubes. What is this: EBP, QI, or research?*

A: Research. The keyword that indicates that this is research is "effective." Research is about reliably determining what is an effective treatment. The question is key. This question is, does cola effectively unclog NG tubes? There is a clear direction that the authors of the question want to see happen. This makes this a research question, not a PICOT question, which is nondirectional. PICOT questions ask how does an intervention affect an outcome, which is without a preconceived outcome. The study proposed here would generate knowledge that would help guide practice versus implementing knowledge into practice. QI is not an option as this is not ongoing monitoring; it is new knowledge generation.

Pulling the Evidence Together: Processes of Each Worldview

Definitions are only part of the understanding of these important worldviews. Each of these worldviews has a specific process that is to be followed to ensure the achievement of outcomes expected by the worldview. The differences among EBP, QI, and research have been discussed over the past several years (Cepero, 2011; Harrison, Mackey, & Friedberg, 2008; Hedges, 2006; Newhouse, 2007; Raines, 2012; Shirey et al., 2011). Consider again the premise that research is *generation of knowledge* about what works. EBP is *translating* that knowledge into a *relevant context*. QI is *monitoring ongoing progress* to determine how well the processes are working to achieve the identified outcomes related to a particular issue (see Table 2.2).

EBP Process

Often, nurses tell me how frustrating it is to engage the EBP process. For example, they have said that PICOT questions don't fit all clinical inquiries; searching is too hard; and appraisal is too daunting (Solomons & Spross, 2011). Given these concerns, there is a tendency to ask

Table 2.2   EBP, QI, and Research Processes

	EBP	QI	Research
Focus	Translating information into practice	Monitoring ongoing care processes and outcomes	Generating new, generalizable knowledge
Method	Seven-step Process: Inquiry to Dissemination	PDSA; FOCUS-PDSA	Quantitative Qualitative Mixed Methods
Persons involved	All who influence a clinical issue (both actively and passively)	Quality decision-makers Unit-level personnel	Researcher Research team Sample
Results	Practice change to sustain impact on outcome	Process change to ensure accuracy of process and outcomes	New knowledge and new understanding of reliable practices
Who should use results	Unit/service line/ organization	Organization	Health care community
Purpose of IRB approval	Use of patient data	Use of patient data	Patient safety and use of patient data

whether or not the EBP process should be followed thoroughly. Although that's a reasonable question, educators and clinicians agree that rigor is a requirement of the research process, and it is the same with the EBP and QI processes. The reliability of outcomes becomes suspect if proper processes are not followed.

The EBP process is comprised of seven steps (see Figure 2.4). Each of these steps is sequential; for example, Step 5 must come after Step 4.

Step 0—Clinical inquiry. The first step is actually step zero, and it comes before all other steps. This step is fostering of clinical inquiry and requires that an issue be meaningful to those who are engaging it. This is sometimes not how change occurs in health care. Rather change can be dictated to those who have to engage it, which does not encourage inquiry or investment in the change process.

Seven-Step EBP Process	
Step 0	Clinical Inquiry
Step 1	Clinical Question
Step 2	Search for Answer from Health Care Database
Step 3	Critical Appraisal of Evidence
Step 4	Implementation of Evidence into Practice
Step 5	Evaluation of Outcome
Step 6	Dissemination of Implementation Results

Figure 2.4   Seven-step EBP process

Step 1—Clinical question. Step 1 is asking the clinical question in a format that will assist clinicians with carefully honing what they really want to know. One such format is PICOT:

P   Population to which the answer will be applied

I   Issue of interest or the intervention that clinicians want to implement

C   Comparison intervention for those questions when *I* is an intervention and is usually what is currently the standard of care

O   Outcome that clinicians want to see changed (for example, patient satisfaction, length of stay, or pressure ulcers)

T   Time it takes for the intervention to achieve the outcome

By their definition, the *C* and *T* are relevant in most, but not all, questions (Fineout-Overholt & Stillwell, 2011).

Step 2—Search for answer from health care databases. A well-constructed PICOT question leads to Step 2, which is finding the answer through systematically searching relevant databases. Searching using the PICOT question components is critical to finding the best answer. Furthermore, searching three health care databases using keywords and controlled vocabulary (e.g., MeSH headings) is required to thoroughly establish that a systematic search has been conducted. Librarians are key partners in Step 2 as they are able to assist clinicians in finding evidence/studies that can help answer the PICOT question. There are several substeps within Step 2 (Fineout-Overholt, Berryman, Hofstetter, & Sollenberger, 2011; Stillwell, Fineout-Overholt, Melnyk, & Williamson, 2010):

1. Including combining keyword and controlled vocabulary searches

2. Applying limits to these subsequent groups of studies

3. Applying inclusion or exclusion criteria to the group of studies that helps further determine which studies in the group will help answer the questions

(See Chapter 6 for more information on finding evidence.)

Identifying Levels of Evidence

There are different levels of evidence to answer PICOT questions (see Table 2.3). You can use an Evidence Hierarchy to identify the level of evidence of articles you have found to answer your PICOT question. Enter the "level" in the column labeled "Strength of the Evidence" on your evaluation/synthesis table.

Table 2.3   Sample Rating System for the Hierarchy of Evidence

Level of Evidence	Sources of Evidence
Level I	Evidence from a systematic review or meta-analysis of all relevant RCTs
Level II	Evidence from well-designed RCTs
Level III	Evidence from well-designed controlled trials without randomization
Level IV	Evidence from well-designed case-control and cohort studies
Level V	Evidence from systematic reviews of descriptive and qualitative studies
Level VI	Evidence from single descriptive or qualitative studies
Level VII	Evidence from the opinion of authorities and/or reports of expert committees

Source: Modified from Melnyk & Fineout-Overholt 2011.

Q: *Our unit has completed a critical appraisal of the literature about a topic of importance to our practice. How do we know when we have enough evidence?*

A: Saturation when searching! If you are repeatedly finding the same articles, you have reached saturation.

Step 3—Critical appraisal of evidence. Step 3 is critical appraisal of the evidence that is in the final group of studies retrieved in Step 2. In Step 3, there are three phases:

1. Rapid critical appraisal, in which studies are evaluated for their validity, reliability and applicability to the patients who generated the clinical question. When these aspects are established, the study becomes a keeper study (a study that is kept for further evaluation) (Fineout-Overholt et al., 2010a, 2010b).

2. Evaluation, which is further analyzing the keeper studies for similarities and differences by placing essential study data in an evaluation table (see Figure 2.5).

3. Synthesis, which is extracting data from the evaluation table for the purpose of distilling down the information into "what we know" about the issue of interest and placing these descriptive data in an informative synthesis table (see Tables 2.6 and 2.7).

The table shown in Figure 2.6 is one example/template for how you could construct a synthesis table focused on comparing interventions across studies.

The table shown in Figure 2.7 is another example/template for a synthesis table focused on comparing study design, sample, and outcome across studies. There could be many more foci for syntheses tables. The point is to create your *own* synthesis table that reflects the story the studies are telling about your issue! Choose carefully your information to include in your syntheses tables so that it is clear to others what the overall message is from your studies.

Step 3 is a critical step that often is challenging to clinicians as it takes time and requires specialized skills in understanding how to determine the quality of research methods and their impact on the usefulness of the research findings to practice (Fineout-Overholt et al., 2010c). The novice researcher should seek assistance of an experienced mentor (e.g., nurse scientist or APN).

Citation: Author(s), date of publication, and title	Conceptual Framework	Design/Method	Sample/Setting	Major Variables Studied and Their Definitions	Measurement of Major Variables	Data Analysis	Study Findings	Strength of the Evidence (i.e., level of evidence + quality [study strengths and weaknesses])
Author, Year, Title	*Theoretical basis for study*		*Number, Characteristics, Attrition rate and why?*	*Independent variables (e.g., IV1 = IV2 =) Dependent variables (e.g., DV =)*	*What scales were used to measure the outcome variables (e.g., name of scale, author, reliability info [e.g., Cronbach alphas])*	*What stats were used to answer the clinical question (i.e, all stats do not need to be put into the table)*	*Statistical findings or qualitative findings (i.e., for every statistical test you have in the data analysis column, you should have a finding)*	*1. Strengths and limitations of the study 2. Risk or harm if study intervention or findings implemented 3. Feasibility of use in your practice 4. Remember: level of evidence + quality of evidence = strength of evidence and confidence to act 5. Use the USPSTF grading schema http://www.ahrq.gov/clinic/3rduspstf/ratings.htm*

Caveats
- The *only studies you should put in these tables are the ones that you know answer your question* after you have done rapid critical appraisal (i.e., the keeper studies).
- Use abbreviations and create a legend for yourself and readers.
- Keep your descriptions brief. There should be NO complete sentences.
- This evaluation is for the purpose of knowing your studies to synthesize.

These italicized terms are prompts to help you with what should be included in these columns.

Used with permission, ©2007 Fineout-Overholt.

Figure 2.5   Evaluation table template

Comparisons of Variable of Interest: Outcome, Intervention, Measurement, Definition of Variable, Levels of Evidence [design] Across Studies

	Studies	A	B	C	D	E	F
Interventions							
1		X	X			X	X
2				X	X		X
3				X	X		X

Legend: A–F would be study author and year; X indicates presence of interventions 1, 2, and/or 3.

Used with permission, ©2007 Fineout-Overholt.

Figure 2.6   Evidence synthesis: Sample 1

Studies	Design	Sample	Outcome

A	RCT	N=450
		Age: 60–90
		Ethnicity:
		  80% Asian
		  20% Caucasian
			Falls ⇩

B	Quasi-experimental, correlational	N=35
		Age: 75–85
		Ethnicity:
		  73% Caucasian
		  10% African American
		  17% Hispanic
			Falls ⇩

C	EBP implementation project	N=50 Age: 55–90 Ethnicity: 100% Caucasian	Falls ⇩

Used with permission, ©2007 Fineout-Overholt.

Figure 2.7   Evidence synthesis: Sample 2

Step 4—Implementation of evidence into practice. Step 4 is taking the best of "what we know" and combining it with internal evidence, your expertise, and patient preferences as you integrate what you now know works into practice. If there is insufficient evidence or the evidence is not well done, then clinicians have the obligation to find an answer through generating knowledge that is generalizable (research) or focused on their agency (QI).

Step 5—Evaluation of outcome. In Step 5, outcomes of integrating the evidence into practice are evaluated. For example, this evaluation could involve a premeasure of outcomes, the evidence-based intervention implementation, and the postmeasure of outcomes.

Step 6—Dissemination of implementation results. Dissemination can range from presentation at the local agency to international presentation to publishing in a peer-reviewed journal. One important caveat about publication of an evidence implementation project is to report the work as a *project* and *not* as a *research study*.

The EBP process is beneficial to improving patient outcomes. When followed closely, the benefits are immeasurable for patients and their families, systems, and providers.

QI Process

The QI process involves rapid cycle testing, referred to earlier as *PDSA*. This rapid cycling offers opportunity to try something to quickly see if it works in a way that facilitates real-time decision-making (Foster & Kosmach, 2009). First you develop a plan to test a new way of delivering care by identifying objectives for the project and predicting the outcome (Plan), which is often generated from ideas of clinicians and may include data from practice. Next, you carry out the test (Do), which involves observing how things go and documenting unexpected outcomes. The next required step is to conduct a discussion about the observed outcomes achieved and what can be learned from them (Study). Finally, the team determines any modifications that need to be made (Act/Adjust) to improve the process (Varkey & Kollengode, 2011).

Research Process

The research process follows very strict rules that cannot be adjusted; otherwise, the results are not credible. There are two approaches to generating research: quantitative and qualitative. Some of the steps of the quantitative research process seem very similar to the EBP and QI processes; however, when researchers conceptualize a research problem (initial step), they are considering it from a different point of view and application than a clinician. In part, this has helped to generate a gap between practice and research. With the increasing use of EBP, this gap is closing as researchers and clinicians are discussing what issues are relevant to improving patient, provider, and system outcomes, and these issues are driving the research generation.

For researchers using quantitative methods, the next step is to determine or develop the conceptual framework that will drive their research. This means that they determine before they start their study how they believe relationships will turn out or what outcome they will achieve and how it will be achieved. This is different from the initial stages of EBP in which the clinician is not sure how the intervention or issue will affect the desired outcome. To that end, clinicians look to the synthesis of the literature to inform them about a particular outcome and its relationship to certain interventions. For researchers, identifying the conceptual framework is critical to the reliability of their work.

> **Q:** *Is the research process for qualitative research any different from the process for quantitative research?*
>
> **A:** The process/approach for qualitative research is different from quantitative research; however, it is not at all less rigorous. There are different approaches to studying different issues within qualitative research. These are described in greater detail in Chapter 12.

After the research problem is considered within the chosen conceptual framework, researchers identify the most appropriate research design that can help resolve the research problem. For example, if a decrease in an untoward outcome is the research problem, then an intervention is the resolution and a randomized controlled trial is the design of choice. This is the strongest research design and the only one that definitively can identify the cause and effect relationship between what you do (i.e., the intervention) and the outcome. There are many research designs that match specific research issues (see Table 2.4 and Chapter 7). The controlled aspect of the trial is when researchers collect data about other influences on the outcome. Taking this step enables researchers to be confident in the relationship between the intervention and the outcome.

Table 2.4   Examples of Types of Research Questions and Associated Research Designs

Research Questions About	Sample Research Designs
Interventions that increase good outcomes/decrease bad outcomes	Randomized Controlled Trial
Conditions associated with outcome	Cohort Study; Case-Control Study
Assessment to improve diagnosis	Randomized Controlled Trial and/or Cohort Study
Interventions to predict impact on outcome	Prospective Study and/or Randomized Controlled Trial
Intervention to reduce known risk for disease or associated outcomes	Cohort Study and/or Case-Control Studies
Human experience	Qualitative Study

After the design is determined, researchers craft their study within the chosen design parameters. Participant safety is a primary concern with any research method, and approval from a participant safety board, often called the *human subjects review board (HSRB)* or *Institutional Review Board (IRB)* must be obtained prior to the initiation of the study. This approval indicates that careful attention has been given to ensure participant safety during the study.

> **Q:** *Is approval from an IRB necessary for EBP, QI, or research processes?*
>
> **A:** Given that participant safety is addressed within the research process, IRB *for participant safety* is not necessary within the EBP or QI process; however review may be necessary to ensure patient information (e.g., chart audit; outcome evaluation) will be treated ethically and the Health Insurance Portability and Accountability Act (HIPAA) is not violated.

Data collection and analysis are key parts of the research process. There are many parameters or rules within these steps that must be followed. The steps in quantitative research enable researchers to determine the effect of the intervention, and the steps in qualitative research assist the researcher in further understanding what is being studied.

Interpreting the study results is one of the final steps in research, and it involves under-standing the data analysis and drawing conclusions about the issue being studied. Research-ers attempt to put the results in a context of the existing literature. Discussion around the results and why they occurred is common. There is also discussion regarding the design, circumstances that occurred during the study, and other aspects of the study that could limit the generalizability and reliability of the study results. After the results have been interpreted, researchers write a scholarly report of the study and publish it for others to learn about what has been done. The "so what" factor for health care research is whether or not it will make a meaningful difference to patient care. Although some researchers may not have the "so what" factor in mind when they conduct their studies, the final step in the research process should be consideration of how the results of the study can be applied to everyday practice.

The Bottom Line: Purposes and Related Outcomes for EBP, QI, and Research

The purposes of EBP, QI, and research help us to further understand the links among these worldviews and their processes. The purpose of EBP is to use the best evidence (internal and external) in making patient care decisions by translating existing knowledge into prac-tice. This purpose culminates in achieving best patient outcomes. The desire for a reliable approach to achieving these outcomes is what drives EBP. Clinicians are interested in estab-lished care delivery methods and interventions versus less reliable, trial-and-error processes that may or may not achieve the desired outcomes. This is why EBP is essential to achieving the best outcomes for individuals, systems, communities, and groups.

The purpose of research is applying a rigorous methodology to discover new knowledge that is applicable to a broad spectrum of patients. This broad application is called *generaliz-ability*. This unique purpose belongs solely to research. Care of an individual patient is not the focus of research. This purpose must be met for external evidence to be useful for EBP. The deciding factor for a "study" to be deemed research is whether it meets the following criteria:

1. Has rigorous systematic research design

2. Generates new knowledge

3. Is generalizable to a broad spectrum of people

The purpose of QI is to determine a system by which to assess and monitor the quality and appropriateness of care. QI tends to focus on the processes that will achieve the desired outcomes as well as the ongoing evaluation of outcomes. The marker for QI is that the knowledge generated from practice data is useful to the organization/agency as ongoing information about how well we're doing!

In considering the purpose and outcomes of each of these worldviews and processes, terminology becomes important for keeping straight these three important aspects that together help clinicians ensure best outcomes for patients. One such term that can present challenges is *study,* which is unique to research. Study implies rigorous use of techniques and methods that will allow for inference (i.e., did the intervention/condition cause the outcome) and generalizability.

QI and EBP do not have studies; rather, the appropriate term for QI and EBP endeavors is *project.* EBP projects are implementing evidence into practice; therefore, using the term *implementation project* is helpful to distinguish them from QI projects. Finally, the term *evidence-based research* is not accurate. Research *is* evidence; therefore, this term is misleading and can be confusing. Using the appropriate term—*research study*, *QI project*, or *EBP implementation project*—will help everyone be clear on what purpose you are fulfilling and what outcomes you can expect from your efforts.

Points of Clarity and Intersection: Outcomes Research, Translational Research, and Implementation Science

Now that you have a clearer understanding of EBP, QI, and research, there are some related methods that are important to address here because you will frequently encounter them as you employ any of the worldviews described in this chapter. Outcomes research, translational research, and implementation science are related to EBP and QI, but they fall into the category of research. Each is a study of different aspects of moving research evidence into practice.

According to the Agency for Healthcare Quality & Research (AHRQ; 2013), outcomes research is the study of how to achieve outcomes that matter to patients. Research may be one step removed from patients' values, but outcomes research offers opportunity to discover *what outcomes are meaningful* to the end user (e.g., patient, family) of a scientifically established intervention (i.e., one that works).

Translational research, according to the National Institutes of Health, is the study of *how to get scientific discoveries into practice applications* (2013). These research findings offer opportunity to improve practice outcomes and offer ideas for future research as well.

Implementation science is conducting research to determine which strategies are the most efficient to get an evidence-based intervention *sustainably* into practice. It also determines what contributes to and detracts from the efficient working of these strategies (Titler, 2008).

Although these aspects of research enhance EBP and QI, they are not substitutes for EBP and QI. Clinicians are responsible for making sure that their patients receive the best care possible—through understanding what is going on in their practices (QI), understanding what practices have been studied (research), and which ones bear implementation into practice because they are meaningful to patients and clinicians can reliably expect to get their associated outcomes (EBP).

Now that you have read about the definitions, processes, and purposes of EBP, QI, and research, which would you say they are—strange bedfellows or kindred spirits? As you ponder your answer, ask yourself two related questions:

- Which worldview will you have when you use these tools to improve patient care outcomes?

- Which worldview would you prefer your health care providers to have when caring for you?

Try It Now!

Think of an issue that you have encountered in your practice (whatever the setting). Ask yourself which approach/worldview do you need to start with to be able to find a solution/answer to the issue: EBP, QI, or research? Outline how these three worldviews interface as you find the solution.

References

AHRQ (2013). Outcomes Research Fact Sheet. Retrieved from http://www.ahrq.gov/research/findings/factsheets/outcomes/outfact/index.html

Cepero, J. (2011). Differences among quality improvement, evidence-based practice, and research. *Journal of Neuroscience Nursing, 43*(4), 230–232.

Deming Model. (1982). Retrieved from http://www.ihi.org/IHI/Topics/Improvement/ImprovementMethods/ HowToImprove/

Deming, W. E. (1982). *Out of the crisis.* Cambridge, MA: Massachusetts Institute of Technology, CAES.

Fineout-Overholt, E., Berryman, D., Hofstetter, S., & Sollenberger, J. (2011). Finding relevant evidence to answer clinical questions. In B. M. Melnyk & E. Fineout-Overholt, *Evidence-based practice in nursing and healthcare: A guide to best practice* (2nd ed.). (pp. 40–70). Philadelphia: Lippincott, Williams & Wilkins.

Fineout-Overholt, E., Melnyk, B. M., Stillwell, S. B., & Williamson, K. M. (2010a). Evidence-based practice step by step: Critical appraisal of the evidence: part I. *American Journal of Nursing, 110*(7), 47–52.

Fineout-Overholt, E., Melnyk, B. M., Stillwell, S. B., & Williamson, K. M. (2010b). Evidence-based practice, step by step: Critical appraisal of the evidence: part II: Digging deeper-examining the "keeper" studies. *American Journal of Nursing, 110*(9), 41–48.

Fineout-Overholt, E., Melnyk, B. M., Stillwell, S. B., & Williamson, K. M. (2010c). Evidence-based practice, step by step: Critical appraisal of the evidence: part III. *American Journal of Nursing, 111*(11), 43–51.

Fineout -Overholt, E. & Stillwell, S. (2011). Asking compelling clinical questions. In B. M. Melnyk & E. Fineout-Overholt's *Evidence-based practice in nursing and healthcare: A guide to best practice* (2nd ed). (pp. 25–39). Philadelphia: Lippincott, Williams & Wilkins.

Foster, J., & Kosmach, S. (2009). Is it research or quality improvement? *Clinical Nurse Specialist, 32*(2), 103.

Harrison, M. B., Mackey, M., & Friedberg, E. (2008). Pressure ulcer monitoring: A process of evidence-based practice, quality, and research. *Joint Commission Journal on Quality and Patient Safety, 34*(6), 355–359.

Hedges C. (2006). Research, evidence-based practice, and quality improvement. *AACN Advanced Critical Care, 17*(4), 457–469.

Lamber, M., & Shearer, M. (2010). Developing a common language for evaluation questions in quality and safety improvement. *Quality & Safety in Health Care, 19*, 266–270.

Marshall, G. (1970-1975). Odd Couple (Comedy). New York, New York: Paramount Network.

Melnyk, B. M., & Fineout-Overholt, E. (2003). EBP paradigm. ARCC Publications: Rochester, NY.

Melnyk, B. M., & Fineout-Overholt, E. (2011). *Evidence-based practice in nursing & healthcare: A guide to best practice.* Philadelphia, PA: Lippincott, Williams & Wilkins.

Montgomery, L. M. (1918). *Anne of Green Gables.* Boston: L.C. Page & Co. Publication.

National Institutes of Health (2013). Translational research. Retrieved from http://commonfund.nih.gov/ clinicalresearch/overview-translational.aspx

Newhouse, R. P. (2007). Diffusing confusion among evidence-based practice, quality improvement and research. *Journal of Nursing Administration, 37*(10), 432–435.

Polit, D. F., & Beck, C. T. (2011). *Nursing research: Generating and assessing evidence of nursing practice* (9th ed.). Philadelphia, PA: Lippincott, Williams & Wilkins.

Raines, D. (2012). Quality improvement, evidence-based practice, and nursing research…oh my! *Neonatal Network, 31*(4), 262–264.

Sackett, D. L., Straus, S. E., Richardson, W. S., Rosenberg, W., & Haynes, R. B. (2000). *Evidence-based medicine: How to practice and teach EBM.* Edinburgh: Churchill Livingstone.

Shirey, M. R., Hauck, S. L., Embree, J. L., Kinner T. J., Schaar, G. L., Phillips, L. A., … McCool, I. A. (2011). Showcasing differences between quality improvement, evidence-based practice, and research. *Journal of Continuing Education in Nursing, 42*(2), 57–68.

Solomons, N. M., & Spross, J. A. (2011). Evidence-based practice barriers and facilitators from a continuous quality improvement perspective: An integrative review. *Journal of Nursing Management, 19,* 109–120.

Stillwell, S. B., Fineout-Overholt, E., Melnyk, B. M., & Williamson, K. M. (2010). Evidence-based practice: Step by step: Searching for the evidence. *American Journal of Nursing, 110*(3), 41–47.

Titler, M. G. (2008). The evidence for evidence-based practice implementation. In R. G. Hughes (Ed.), *Patient safety and quality: An evidence-based handbook for nurses* (Chapter 7). Rockville, MD: Agency for Healthcare Research and Quality (US).

Varkey, P., & Kollengode, A. (2011). A framework for healthcare quality improvement in India: The time is here and now! *Journal of Postgraduate Medicine, 57*(3), 237–241.

Reading and Conducting Research "Head to Toe"

II

"The journey of a thousand miles begins with a single step. Let your journey begin."

–Chinese philosopher Lao-tzu

Getting Started: Finding Ideas for Research

3

Marianne Chulay

WHAT YOU'LL LEARN IN THIS CHAPTER

- Your own clinical experience is a good place to start for research ideas.

- Myriad other resources can help you find a good research idea.

- Good potential research questions have important characteristics that you should adhere to when devising your question.

- A formal rating process will help you to objectively evaluate your potential research study.

After you have a strong supportive research infrastructure in place, you can begin to think about topics for research studies. The first step in the research journey is to identify a topic for a research study. Of all the steps in the research process, none could be more important than finding a good research idea that can lead to a potential research question. If you rush through this beginning step without making sure you select a research question appropriate to your practice situation that is feasible for conduct by clinicians and important to patient care, you could go down a path that will make completion of your research journey difficult or impossible.

This chapter provides information to help you identify an appropriate research topic. The chapter starts with information on different processes or places that nurses can use to generate a list of potential research ideas or questions. Then, the chapter describes a rating process that will help you determine which of the ideas or potential questions would be best suited for your clinical project.

Where to Find Research Ideas

Research ideas abound, and you can find research ideas in a number of ways. Approaches range from examining your clinical practice situation to reviewing a list of research priorities identified by experts or nursing organizations. This section describes both approaches in detail.

Clinical Experience as a Source of Research Ideas

A good place to begin your search for a research idea is to examine your current clinical practice situation. This approach helps you identify questions that are most likely to be relevant and meaningful to patient care on your unit (Burns, 2001; Chulay, 1997; Chulay, 2006). For example, nurses on a labor and delivery unit might use two different methods to support mothers during the second stage of labor and wonder which one is superior. Or on a cardiology unit with most patients on telemetry, a nurse might question whether skin preparation before placing electrodes makes a difference in electrode adherence. Next, we describe a strategy for not only identifying such topics, but also narrowing these topics down into potential research questions.

For some nurses, starting with a potential research question may be intimidating. One simple strategy to help nurses find potential research questions, called the *Focus Group Method*, is to hold several brief meetings on the unit to identify clinical practice issues of importance to bedside nurses (Campbell & Chulay, 1990; Chulay, 2001; Chulay, 2006; Granger & Chulay, 1999). After topics of importance have been articulated, you can identify those that are conducive to being researched. Asking someone to serve as the focus group leader will facilitate productivity at the sessions. Anyone with experience leading groups, such as advanced practice nurses or clinical educators, could serve as a focus group leader.

> **Q:** *How can I encourage interest and participation in focus group meetings?*
>
> **A:** Limiting the work in the first few sessions to tasks that are easy for nurses to complete will encourage active participation by all attendees. Putting the focus on improving patient care, rather than research, will help avoid intimidation of nurses who have never done research.

To begin the focus group meeting, ask nurses to brainstorm a list of common patient care problems, as well as nursing interventions that staff perform multiple times each day. Providing five or six major categories relating to their practice will help nurses more thoroughly consider their nursing practice. Some examples include:

- Patient populations/diagnosis/reason for admission/age/comorbidities
- Patient problems
- Common symptoms managed by nurses
- Nursing interventions
- Important patient outcomes to be achieved at transfer/discharge
- Common equipment used to provide patient care

When you've compiled a list, it will paint a vivid picture of the nurses' everyday practice, making it easier for them to brainstorm clinical questions. Without this foundation, nurses may not only underestimate the breadth of their everyday practice, but also tend to focus on clinical practice issues that, although challenging, are not seen or experienced every day on their unit. (As will be discussed later in this chapter, a key to a successful research study for nurses is identifying an issue or problem that is present every day in their practice.)

In the second step of the Focus Group Method, ask nurses to raise clinical questions about items on their list of high-volume problems and nursing interventions. Nurses are encouraged to question items on the high-volume list by asking questions such as:

- "What is the best way to do *X*?"
- "Is there a more efficient way to do *Y*?"
- "Does *Z* really improve patient care?"

The emphasis in this step is on *clinical* questions, not *research* questions. Some of the questions raised may be answered through a quality improvement (QI) or evidence-based practice (EBP) project and not require research. (Chapter 2 outlined the differences between EBP, QI, and research.) In a typical one-hour session, nurses should be able to quickly identify a list of common patient care issues as well as 10 to 20 clinical questions.

For example, in a list compiled by oncology nurses, pharmacologic and nonpharmacologic management of nausea and pain would likely be listed under the category of common nursing interventions. As the clinicians begin brainstorming clinical questions, they would be encouraged to raise questions about the best way to nonpharmacologically manage nausea. Several clinical questions would likely emerge from the participants based on different approaches used to manage nausea that continues when pharmacologic interventions are not adequate.

In the next meeting, the list of clinical questions can be narrowed down to five or six by having participants eliminate questions that are not *clinically* interesting or not important to patient care from their perspective. A fun way to accomplish this process is to list all the questions on a flip chart and ask everyone to vote on which questions should be discarded. You can give each participant "sticky dots" to place next to the questions he or she wants to vote off the list to make this a more fun (and potentially chaotic) method to eliminate questions. (See "Critical Evaluation of Potential Research Questions" later in this chapter.)

 What makes a question clinically interesting?

 A question is clinically interesting if it is derived from questions nurses ask about their everyday practice.

When the voting is done, the remaining questions will represent clinical practice questions of high interest to the staff. You can then critically evaluate the questions to determine which ones would be appropriate and feasible to be addressed as potential research questions.

Other Sources of Research Ideas

A number of other sources could also be of help to finding research questions or ideas for studies. Other sources of research ideas include the following:

- Information from organizational data

- Listings of nursing research priorities

- Suggestions for further study in published research

- Journal clubs

These sources, including their advantages, are described next.

Information from organizational data. One source of potential research questions is data generated from organizational activities targeted to improve patient care quality. For example, the data from QI projects or the monitoring of quality indicators can help identify patient care situations that require further improvement (see Chapter 2). Other organizational data sources include EBP projects and results of patient care surveys. Final reports from these organizational initiatives often include suggestions for practice change or recommendations for research studies. You can use these recommendations to generate potential research questions.

Listings of nursing research priorities. Based on their perspective of what areas of nursing practice need further study, national nursing associations or specialty nurse experts sometimes generate lists of nursing research priorities. These lists are then either published in nursing journals and/or listed on websites of professional nursing organizations. For example, the Emergency Nurses Association lists on its website specific practice research priorities in the broad categories of emergency department overcrowding and boarding, psychiatric emergencies, and workplace violence. The American Association of Critical-Care Nurses lists broad areas of patient care that need additional research, including effective and appropriate use of technology to achieve optimal patient assessment, management, and/or outcomes; creation of a healing environment; and prevention and management of complications of critical illness. The following list includes several sources for listings of nursing research priorities for specialty nursing practice areas:

- "ONS Research Priorities Survey" in *Oncology Nursing Forum* (Doorenbos et al., 2008).

- "Neurocritical Care Nursing Research Priorities" in *Neurocritical Care* (Olson, et al., 2012).

- "Research Council Co-Chairs Publish on Psychiatric Nursing Research Priorities" in *Journal of the American Psychiatric Nurses Association* (Willis, Beeber, Mahoney, & Sharp, 2011).

- "Developing Military Nursing Research Priorities" in *Military Medicine* (Duong et al., 2005).

- American Association of Critical-Care Nurses research priorities: http://www.aacn.org/wd/practice/content/research/research-priority-areas.pcms?menu=practice

- American Heart Association Council on Cardiovascular and Stroke Nursing research priorities: http://my.americanheart.org/professional/Councils/CVN/Council-on-Cardiovascular-and-Stroke-Nursing_UCM_320474_SubHomePage.jsp

- National Association of Orthopedic Nurses research priorities: http://www.orthonurse.org/p/cm/ld/fid=48

- Oncology Nursing Society research priorities: http://www.ons.org/Research#agenda

- Emergency Nurses Association research priorities: http://www.ena.org/IENR/priorities/Pages/Default.aspx

Using listings of research priorities to identify a potential question has the advantage of being an easy way to find questions. Even though the questions on these lists are considered high priority for study by experts in nursing, it will be especially important for nurses to evaluate if the questions are actually appropriate and feasible for their clinical practice (see "Critical Evaluation of Potential Research Questions" later in this chapter). The mere presence of a question on one of these lists often indicates that other researchers, likely with much more research experience than the average nurse possesses, have not found the method or resources to do the study themselves.

Suggestions for further study in published research. The "Conclusion" section of published research studies, reviews of the literature, and articles by content experts often list a number of ideas for future research. Authors typically suggest circumstances under which previous studies need to be repeated (i.e., in different patient populations or age groups) or the next studies that need to be done to advance understanding of the research area.

The advantage of finding potential research questions from published sources is that the suggested questions are coming from individuals with a strong background or expertise in the topic area. As previously mentioned, however, it is important to evaluate whether the suggested questions or ideas for future research are appropriate for nurses to conduct in their own clinical practice. (See "Critical Evaluation of Potential Research Questions" later in this chapter.)

Q: *I just found out that my potential research question has already been addressed in previously published research? What do I do now?*

A: First, and foremost, it is important to know that a single study on any topic is unlikely to provide a definitive answer on how best to provide patient care in all circumstances. Repeating studies is important to truly understanding clinical phenomenon. Later in the chapter, a variety of different ways to repeat studies is described.

Journal clubs. Journal clubs are another frequently suggested source for generating potential questions for research studies (Berger, Hardin, & Topp, 2011; Luby, Riley, & Towne, 2006; Polit & Beck, 2012; Silversides, 2011). A journal article is selected for review by interested participants prior to the journal club meeting. Good articles are those in which the studies pertain to those clinical practice issues commonly encountered on your unit. For example, a study on the administration of a topical anesthetic to prevent pain associated with insertion of an intravenous device would be a good article if this is a regular part of your practice. Ideas for additional research studies can be either to replicate the journal club study (see later content) or use one of the ideas for future research identified by the study investigators in the "Discussion" section.

While journal clubs have the potential to identify research questions/ideas, their success is often limited by a number of challenges, such as poor meeting attendance, poor compliance with reading the article in advance of the meeting, and/or limited emphasis in the meeting discussion on future research needs. Also, research questions identified in the journal club may not be relevant to your patient care situation, which is an important criteria for a good research study.

Characteristics of Good Research Questions

No matter the source of the potential research question, it is critical that you determine its appropriateness and feasibility for a study by nurses (Chulay, 2001; Chulay, 2006; Granger & Chulay, 1999). Although a research question might be recommended by experts or sound like a great study, it may not be a good research study for novice nurse researchers. Unlike individuals in academic positions, frontline nurses have limited time and resources for engaging in research activities. Taking time to evaluate whether the potential question meets the criteria of a good research study will avoid questions that are beyond the scope of the nurse researcher or available resources. Better to find out early that a question you love is actually too difficult for you to study at this particular time than to make the discovery after investing months of work on the project before you encounter roadblocks to completing the study.

To assure selection of an appropriate question for a research study, you should evaluate proposed questions against criteria of a good study. It is important to note that these criteria are different from criteria that might be used for academic research projects (i.e., thesis or dissertation topics; faculty research). Characteristics of a good study for frontline nurses include:

- Replication study (previous research exists which could be repeated)

- Quick and easy data collection

- Large number of eligible patients

- Large sample size not required

- Additional funds not required

- Within nursing control

- Availability of methods to measure study outcomes

- Strong interest in topic

- Clinical expertise in topic

- Importance to clinical practice/patient outcomes

- Potential financial impact

It's not necessary that your study include all of these characteristics, but the more characteristics the study meets, the easier it will be to conduct the study and the more likely your study will be completed in a reasonable time frame.

Q: *In general, are there topics that are not considered good research ideas or questions for clinicians?*

A: Yes. Research ideas or questions that require large sample sizes should be avoided. Studies about trying to decrease a currently low incidence or rate of a patient care problem (problems that occur in less than 10% of patients) typically require hundreds of patients in the study. For example, most hospital-acquired infections (ventilator-associated pneumonia, blood stream catheter-related infections, sepsis, methicillin-resistant staphylococcus aureus infections, or vancomycin-resistant infections), hospital-acquired pressure ulcers, prevention of falls, and/or prevention of deep vein thrombosis require sample sizes in the hundreds, if not thousands, of patients. Although these are all important aspects of care that require new approaches to prevent their occurrence, the sample size requirements would likely dictate the need for a multicenter study and years of data collection.

Replication Study

A good research study for you to conduct as a frontline nurse would be to repeat a study that was previously done in the same patient population that you care for on a daily basis. Replication research is the deliberate repetition of research procedures in a second investigation for the purpose of determining if earlier results can be repeated (Connelly, 1986; Polit & Beck, 2012), to overcome flaws or limitations in prior research, or to broaden the validity of the findings for wider application. An advantage of repeating a study done by others is that it enables you to be guided in the design of your study by those who have successfully completed a research study, which is helpful if you have little prior research experience.

Q: *In school, the emphasis was on finding ideas or questions that had not been studied before. Is this a good idea?*

A: For nurses who have little or no experience conducting research, conducting a replication study will result in less time and less frustration in developing the study. Novel research ideas, although intriguing, can require more time and expertise than is available to experientially young researchers, especially those who are trying to do research with the time challenges of a clinical setting. When nurses are oriented to a new practice area, their patient care assignments usually begin with the predictable, least complex patient on the unit and then gradually escalate to the unpredictable, complex patient. Similarly, the types of research studies you tackle should begin with the simpler, more predictable studies rather than a study that has never been done before.

Replication studies are critically important in a practice discipline because they help to establish the validity, or truth, of prior research (Beck, 1994; Blair, 1985; Connelly, 1986; Gould, 2002; Polit & Beck, 2012; Savel & Munro, 2012; Zachariah, 1995). When others are unable to replicate the findings of a study it may:

- Raise questions about the veracity of the prior study

- Indicate that the methods are too complex to be carried out by others or nonexperts

- Indicate that the unique circumstances of the previous study don't apply to other clinical situations

A recent example that underscores the importance of replication to confirm study findings is the removal from the market of a drug to treat sepsis after several studies were unable to achieve similar results to the original, multicenter research study (Savel & Munro, 2012). Replication studies guard against implementation of fraudulent or spurious research findings.

Repetition of studies also allows the findings of the study to be extended to different populations and/or clinical situations. You should not assume that because one study found an intervention or approach to be beneficial in one clinical situation that the intervention will have similar results in a different situation. For example, a study that finds temporal artery thermometers to be accurate in medical, adult patients with normothermic temperatures doesn't mean that similar results will occur when using the device in hypothermic patients. Medical devices that measure physiologic functions rarely perform as well in the extreme ranges of the parameter as in the normal physiologic ranges, so accuracy studies need to be done in a variety of physiologic conditions.

There are a number of ways to perform replication studies (see Table 3.1). Using the same patient population, study design, and study procedures as the prior study is one approach to repeating a study. Other approaches involve altering some aspect of the study to determine which patients are likely to benefit from the intervention. You can repeat the study with a different age group or patient population, with study procedures that are more similar to your clinical practice routines, or with procedures that improve on less than ideal procedures in the prior study.

Table 3.1   Different Types of Replication Studies

Type of Replication	Explanation	Study Example	Value
Exact Duplication	Use of the same, or approximately the same, materials and methods for the replication of the study—study design, subjects, interventions, and procedures.	Replication of an original study that evaluated accuracy of pulmonary artery pressures at different head of bed elevations in cardiac surgical patients. Replication study done with similar materials and methods.	Provides evidence of reliability of the original study and increases confidence in the generalizability of the findings.

Type of Replication	Explanation	Study Example	Value
Constructive Duplication	Tests the relationships established in a prior study, but some aspects of the study methods are deliberately altered (setting, patient population, intervention tested, improvement in study design).	Original studies on pain associated with intravenous catheter insertion measured pain associated with the catheter insertion itself only and not with application of the topical anesthetic. Replication studies improved on the design by also measuring pain with the subcutaneous injection of lidocaine before IV insertion.	Extends the generalizability of the original study findings to new populations, settings, or interventions.
		Original studies evaluated discharge education after cardiac surgery. Replication studies evaluated discharge instruction in patients with chronic heart failure.	
		Original studies evaluated impact of ICU visitation on family member anxiety. Replication studies evaluated impact of PACU visitation on family member anxiety.	
		Original studies evaluated the effect of manual delivery of hyperoxygenation before and after endotracheal suctioning on arterial blood gases. Replication studies evaluated mechanical delivery of the hyperoxygenation intervention.	

continues

Table 3.1   Different Types of Replication Studies   *continued*

Type of Replication	Explanation	Study Example	Value
Operational Duplication	Use of the same, or approximately the same, materials and methods for the replication of the study, but improves on statistical analyses.	Original studies on the accuracy of noninvasive temperature devices used correlational statistics for analysis. Replication study done with similar materials and methods except data analysis did not use correlational tests but calculated bias and precision values and used Bland Altman graphs.	Updates findings using currently accepted statistical methods to either verify or refute prior findings.

Source: Beck, 1994; Connelly, 1986; Polit & Beck, 2012.

Despite the importance of replication studies, some nurse researchers are reticent to conduct this type of study. Their reticence might stem from a need to conduct original research to meet university requirements or to be eligible for research grants. Although the conduct of original research is important to the profession of nursing, so, too, is the replication of those studies to advance our scientific basis for nursing practice.

Quick and Easy Data Collection

Also important when trying to identify an ideal research study is to select a study that enables busy nurses to perform data collection quickly and easily. In most organizations, nurses have to incorporate data collection into their usual care routines—hospital budgets do not usually include funds to pay for staff to collect data. So, data collection must be "doable" by nurses in their usual practice situation, which means the time for data collection on each study participant needs to be no more than 10 to 15 minutes at a time. When you need to collect data, you will likely hand off your patient care assignment to another nurse on the unit so you can focus on data collection. Asking colleagues to take responsibility for your patients for 15 minutes or less may not lead to refusals; however, asking for an hour or more of coverage time isn't likely to be met with enthusiasm.

Studies that require you to collect data at multiple points in time or from participants who are not on your clinical unit are much more difficult to accomplish than studies in which you collect data at one or two time points and when participants are on your unit. An example of a study that strongly meets these criteria is an accuracy study of automated blood pressures (BP) in patients with irregular rhythms. Device BP and heart rates were obtained once for each participant at a time when therapeutic vital signs were required, so the time to add on the second set of research BP and heart rate determination, using the clinical "gold standard" comparison method, was less than 5 minutes. The total time the nurse was away from his/her own patient care responsibilities was less than 10 minutes. An example of a study that did not meet these criteria was one that involved obtaining patient satisfaction ratings with their perioperative experience after the patient had left the perioperative area. Nurses were often gone from their patient care responsibilities for an hour while trying to track down patients on the various surgical floors to get the survey completed.

Large Number of Eligible Patients

When the study to be conducted has eligibility criteria that relate to a large number of patients normally cared for on a unit, the time to complete the study is dramatically shorter than if only some unit patients meet the criteria. In order to complete data collection in a reasonable amount of time (less than 3 months), it is important that the topic of the study be something that relates to at least one patient on the unit every day of the year. That way, even if some eligible patients decide not to participate, which is likely to happen, there should still be enough participating patients to get data collection done in a reasonable amount of time. If nurses have as their goal to enroll one patient per day into the study, then it is possible to complete enrollment of participants in less than 3 months. It is difficult to maintain enthusiasm for research when data collection drags on for 6 months or longer.

For example, nurses working on a cardiology unit who choose to conduct a study that requires patients to have a medical diagnosis of cardiomyopathy would not likely be able to enroll a different patient each day. However, if they conduct a study that requires patients to have a medical diagnosis of myocardial ischemia, they would likely be able to enroll one or more patients each day. Similarly, if they plan a study to evaluate temporal artery thermometers in febrile conditions, then conducting that study in a postanesthesia care unit could conceivably take years. If the study is conducted on a medical unit, it could easily be completed in less than 3 months.

Large Sample Size Not Required

It is essential to know in advance of selecting a potential research question the approximate number of participants required for the study. If the requirement is for more than 75 subjects, you, as a frontline nurse, would be well advised not to embark on that study. The time to complete enrollment in a study that requires 125 or more participants will automatically require data collection to far exceed a few months. Even if more than one patient per day fits the eligibility criteria of a study, it is unrealistic to think that busy nurses would have enough extra time each day to collect data on more than one participant. Although it's theoretically possible to do so with four or five participants a day, the clinical reality is that it would be unlikely to occur. Only rarely is the time for data collection so short that more than one participant could be enrolled each day in the study.

Q: *How do I determine what the sample size needs to be for my study?*

A: Most nurses will need to consult with someone with research expertise to know what an approximate sample size would likely be for their study (see Chapter 8 for additional information on sample size determination). Doctorally prepared nurses, faculty in the school of nursing, and statisticians should have the skills necessary to help with obtaining reasonable estimates of sample sizes.

Additional Funds Not Required

The ideal study does not require any funding by other sources in order to be completed. Noninstitutional research grants are available to help support nursing research, but it is unlikely that someone with limited or no research experience would receive significant funding. The limited number of grants, coupled with the large number of experienced researchers competing for funding, limits the probability that inexperienced researchers will be successful in securing outside funding. So, until you gain more experience with conducting research, you would be wise to focus on studies that do not require large amounts of outside funding.

Although most nursing research budgets have little or no money allocated to fund studies, most nursing administrators would be able to support a study if all that was necessary was a couple hundred dollars to buy research supplies or inexpensive pieces of equipment. This is particularly true if the question to be answered by the study has the potential to improve an important aspect of patient care and if it aligns with organizational priorities. For example, a study that would evaluate pain levels and patient satisfaction with a nonpharmacologic intervention for pain management might require $100 to pay a user fee to use a valid and reliable tool to measure anxiety. Given the importance of the study objective, and its alignment with organizational goals to improve pain management and patient satisfaction, most nursing administrators would likely be able to find funds within the nursing budget to support the user fee.

Within Nursing Control

Many research questions that nurses formulate involve the support of other disciplines to conduct the study. For example, nurses in a postanesthesia care unit might wonder if the use of a particular analgesic would be better at managing postoperative pain than the currently prescribed medications. This might be a great study, but because you do not have the authority to independently order a different postoperative analgesic, you would need to partner with physicians in order to make changes based on your research (see Chapter 5 to learn more about forming research teams). The ideal question for nurses who are independently conducting the research would be one that is within their scope of practice.

Availability of Methods to Measure Study Outcomes

It is important whenever possible to use existing instruments to measure the outcome variable. Even experienced researchers shy away from study topics when measurement of the outcome variable requires them to develop a measurement tool of their own, as explained in Chapter 9.

Strong Interest in Topic

Although it is important to select a study based on organizational priorities (e.g., falls reduction or medication reconciliation) or suggestions by others, it is not usually sufficient. A good research question should also be something you have a strong interest in addressing; otherwise you will lose interest in the project before it is completed. If you do not have a strong interest in the topic, it could be easy to just let the research study die a peaceful death when it doesn't move along as swiftly as you predicted or if you encounter challenges along the way.

Expertise in Topic

Without expertise in the topic, your naiveté might lead you to ask questions that are not relevant or appropriate for study. Another reason this criteria is important is that without expertise in the topic, it might take you longer to develop the study because you will first have to learn about a new area of practice. This criterion is particularly relevant for experientially young researchers—they have enough to learn about how to conduct research without adding to their to-do lists the need to learn about a new topic area.

Importance to Clinical Practice/Patient Outcomes

As already stated, good research studies for nurses are those that are important to clinical practice or patient outcomes. Not only is this type of study more likely to keep your interest throughout the time required to complete the study, but it also helps you to get administrative buy-in and support for the study. If you need a few extra dollars to purchase equipment, or some support needs to be obtained to facilitate data collection, administrative support would come more readily for a study evaluating ways to improve pain management than one that is surveying nurses about uniform preferences.

Potential Financial Impact

The ideal nursing research study has the potential to save the organization money. Savings might occur by simplifying or eliminating care routines (e.g., decreasing supplies or personnel time), improving patient outcomes, or decreasing complications that have fiscal implications (e.g., decreasing length of stay or increasing patient satisfaction). Although not all studies can meet this criteria, its presence is a definite plus, particularly if administrative support to conduct the study is helpful or necessary.

Special Considerations for Neophyte Researchers

When it comes to researchers with little or no prior experience conducting research in the clinical setting (aka neophyte researchers), there are a few additional criteria for a good research question. If you have little research experience, you should not attempt to embark on a research journey without getting someone with research experience to mentor you. Just as you would not allow a new nurse to be oriented to a new clinical practice area without a preceptor, so, too, you should not allow a neophyte researcher to conduct research without a mentor. Individuals who might be able to mentor neophyte researchers include advanced practice nurses, directors of nursing research, research coordinators, faculty at schools of nursing, and/or other nurses who already have extensive research experience.

Another suggestion if you are inexperienced in research is to make sure your research question is narrow in scope to allow the study to be completed as quickly and easily as possible. For example, preventing malnutrition in the hospitalized patient may be the desire, but for neophyte clinical researchers, a research question related to malnutrition would be too broad. Narrowing the question to focus on early identification of at-risk patients for malnutrition would be doable. (Chapter 5 provides information on how to narrow the scope of a research question.)

Another criteria for a good research question for you, as a neophyte researcher, is to avoid overly complex studies. One way to do this is to keep the number of variables in the study to two or three at the most. Even though it might be great to compare five different topical anesthetics for reducing pain of intravenous catheter insertion, it would be wise to study the two methods that are likely to be the most effective in pain reduction for a first study. Then, depending on the study results, other methods could be evaluated in future studies.

Another way to keep studies relatively simple and easy to conduct is to avoid those that require data collection on multiple days from each participant or data collection before or after the patient is on your unit.

Critical Evaluation of Potential Research Questions

Before committing to a research study, it is essential that you carefully determine if the proposed research topic is feasible for study in your clinical practice situation. Using the criteria of a good research study, you can objectively evaluate each potential question by using a formal rating process (see Figure 3.1). Including this step in the final selection of a research study will help you avoid unanticipated roadblocks to study completion. Using a grid with the criteria for a good research study listed in the left column will assure a thorough evaluation and allow easy comparison if more than one question is under consideration.

Evaluation Criteria for Consideration of Clinical Questions for a Research Project

Directions: Rate each clinical question under consideration for a research project/study against the criteria in the left hand column with a number from 0 (criteria not present at all) to 5 (criteria extremely present).

Scoring System (0 to 5 scale): 0 = Criteria not present   5 = Criteria highly present

Criteria of a Good Research Study for Clinicians	First Question	Second Question	Third Question
Topic of interest to clinicians			
Clinicians have clinical expertise in topic area			
Important to clinical practice and/or patient outcomes			
Large number of patients eligible for study (at least 1 new/different patient per day)*			
No political landmines (score as a 5 for topics with no political landmines; 0 for topics with any landmines)*			
Sample size required for study is less than 75 subjects (score as a 5 for questions requiring a sample size of 20 subjects; score as a 3 for questions requiring a sample size of 50 subjects; score as a 0 for topics requiring more than 75 subjects)*			
Clinicians have control over the practice that is to be evaluated in the study (score either a 5 for yes or a 0 for no)*			
Potential financial impact for hospital			
No additional money required (score either as a 5 for questions which would require no money or score as a 0 for questions which require more than $300 in equipment, supplies, etc.)*			
Measurement tools available*			
Data collection for the project would fit with unit routines, not require more than 10 to 15 minutes at time for data collection, and could be finished quickly			
Replication study (score as either a 5 for yes or a 0 for no)			
Total Score			

*A score of 0 on any of these criteria indicates the question is not amendable to a research study at this time by clinicians who have limited research experience.

Used with permission from Marianne Chulay.

Figure 3.1   Scoring sheet to be used for rating individual research ideas against the criteria of a good research study for clinicians.

Refining the Question

After you have selected the potential question for the study, you should refine the question prior to embarking on the next steps in development of the study. When reviewing your question, you should list all the outcome variables, as well as the specific intervention to be evaluated. A helpful way to address this step is to review the research questions or purposes stated in one or two published studies that are similar to the one you are considering. This should give you a good idea of how other researchers have articulated their study questions or purposes.

Some published studies do not explicitly state their research question but have a research purpose statement, which is merely a declarative statement of the study question. For example, when reviewing a prior study on a nonpharmacologic intervention to manage nausea, you would see that the stated purpose of the study was to determine if aromatherapy (three to four whiffs of an alcohol prep pad placed under the nose) is as effective as ondansetron administration to decrease nausea in the postanesthesia patients. If the phrasing of your original question is not as specific (i.e., "Can nausea be decreased with nonpharmacologic interventions?" or "Is aromatherapy effective in treating nausea?") as that stated in the published study, you will have a better understanding of how your question should be rephrased so it is more specific and clear. (Chapter 4 provides information to help you refine and clarify the idea or question you have selected for study.)

Try It Now!

Complete the focus group brainstorming exercise discussed in this chapter, identifying items for each of the categories listed, and then brainstorm clinical questions you might have about items on your high-volume listing.

References

American Association of Critical-Care Nurses research priorities. Retrieved from http://www.aacn.org/wd/practice/content/research/research-priority-areas.pcms?menu=practice

American Heart Association Council on Cardiovascular and Stroke Nursing research priorities. Retrieved from http://my.americanheart.org/professional/Councils/CVN/Council-on-Cardiovascular-and-Stroke-Nursing_UCM_320474_SubHomePage.jsp

Beck, C. T. (1994). Replication strategies for nursing research. *IMAGE: Journal of Nursing Scholarship, 26*(3), 191-194.

Berger, J., Hardin, H., & Topp, R. (2011). Implementing a virtual journal club in a clinical nursing setting. *Journal of Nurses Staff Development*, May-June *27*(3), 116-120.

Blair, C. (1985). The importance of replication of clinical nursing research. *Journal of New York State Nurses Association*, *16*(2), 10-11.

Burns, S. (2001). Clinical research is part of what we do. *Critical Care Nurse*, *22*(2), 100-113.

Campbell, G., & Chulay, M. (1990). Establishing a clinical nursing research program. In J. Spicer & M. Robinson (Eds.), *Environmental management in critical care nursing* (pp. 52-60). Baltimore, MD: Williams & Wilkins.

Chulay, M. (1997). Bridging the research-practice gap. *Critical Care Nurse*, *17*(1), 81-85.

Chulay, M. (2001). Clinician involvement in critical care research. *Critical Care Nursing Clinics of North America*, *13*(1), 53-62.

Chulay, M. (2006). Good research questions for clinicians. *AACN Advanced Critical Care, 17*(3), 253-265.

Connelly, C. (1986). Replication research in nursing. *International Journal of Nursing Studies, 23(1)*, 71-77.

Doorenbos, A. Z., Berger, A. M., Brohard-Holbert, C., Eaton, L., Kozachik, S., LoBiondo-Wood, G. ... Varricchio, C. (2008). ONS research priorities survey. *Oncology Nursing Forum*, *35*(6), E100-107.

Duong, D. N., Schempp, C., Barker, E., Cupples, S., Pierce, P., Ryan-Wenger, N., ... Young-McCaughan, S. (2005). Developing military nursing research priorities. *Military Medicine*, *170*(5), 362-365.

Emergency Nurses Association research priorities. Retrieved from http://www.ena.org/IENR/priorities/Pages/Default.aspx

Gould, D. (2002). Using replication studies to enhance nursing research. *Nursing Standard*, *16*(49), 33-36.

Granger, B., & Chulay, M. (1999). *Research strategies for clinicians*. Stamford, CT: Appleton & Lange.

Luby, M., Riley, J. K., & Towne, G. (2006). Nursing research journal clubs: Bridging the gap between practice and research. *Medsurg Nursing*, *15*(2), 100-102.

National Association of Orthopedic Nurses research priorities. Retrieved from http://www.orthonurse.org/p/cm/ld/fid=48

Olson, D. M., McNett, M. M., Livesay, S., Le Roux, P. D., Suarez, J. I., & Bautista, C. (2012). Neurocritical care nursing research priorities. *Neurocritical Care*, *16*(1), 55-62.

Oncology Nursing Society research priorities. Retrieved from http://www.ons.org/Research#agenda

Polit, D., & Beck, C. (2012). *Essentials of nursing research: Appraising evidence for nursing practice*, (9th ed.). Philadelphia, PA: Lippincott, Williams, & Wilkins.

Savel, R. H., & Munro, C. L. (2012). Evidence-based backlash: The tale of drotrecogin alfa. *American Journal of Critical Care*, *21*(2), 81-83.

Silversides, A. (2011). Journal clubs: A forum for discussion and professional development. *Canadian Nurse, 107*(2), 18-23.

Willis, D. G., Beeber, L. S., Mahoney, J., & Sharp, D. (2011). Research council co-chairs publish on psychiatric nursing research priorities. *Journal of the American Psychiatric Nurses Association, 17*(4), 273.

Zachariah, R. (1995). Re: replication research in nursing. *Research in Nursing and Health, 18*(6), 575-576.

"Life is like a nondirectional hypothesis; you never know in what direction you will end until you are finished."

–Jane Bliss-Holtz

From Idea to Research Question to Hypothesis

4

Jane Bliss-Holtz

WHAT YOU'LL LEARN IN THIS CHAPTER

- Attention needs to be paid to the factors of variables, populations, and feasibility if a strong research question is to be developed.

- Determining the purpose of your study will help you better define what is to be accomplished and how you might go about performing the study.

- Turning your research question into a formal research hypothesis is an important part of the research process.

Benner (1984) noted that the more experience that nurses have, the more likely they are to almost intuitively focus on the most important aspects of a patient's condition that need to be addressed. This process includes being able to ask the right clinical questions that will produce the necessary data on which to base appropriate care. Being able to formulate an appropriate research question (or *problem statement*, as it is sometimes called) is similar to this, as a focused research question and associated research hypotheses will assist you in narrowing down all of the possible research designs, procedures, and measurements. An appropriate research question also enables you to plan and implement a viable research project. This chapter describes the components of a research question and how to formulate the related study purpose and possible research hypotheses.

PICOT Questions and Research Questions: What Is the Difference?

Chapter 3 described the process of generating clinical questions, including how to prioritize and narrow the focus of the clinical topic using the PICOT format, which is an acronym that stands for

Population-Intervention-Comparison/Control-Outcome-Time. Of the four types of clinical questions typically framed in PICOT format—therapy, diagnosis, prognosis, and etiology—questions related to therapy are the most frequently seen (Huang, Lin, & Demner-Fushman, 2006). However, use of PICOT format in *any* of these four types yields the most successful results when the literature is searched for evidence on which to base practice (Schardt, Adams, Owens, Keitz, & Fontelo, 2007).

> **Q:** *If I develop a PICOT question, then why do I need to bother formulating a research question?*
>
> **A:** The process of developing and refining PICOT questions is specific to performing literature searches. PICOT questions alone will not guide the generation of research hypotheses and, subsequently, lead to development of a research study.

You could think of formulating the PICOT question and searching the literature as the early steps of the evidence-based practice (EBP) process. These steps enable you to determine the significance of your clinical topic to your organization and to obtain the best possible yield when literature is searched for existing evidence (Straus, Glasziou, Richardson, & Haynes, 2011). After searching the evidence using a PICOT question and then appraising the evidence, you can determine whether there is enough evidence on which to safely and effectively base your practice.

As I have said to staff nurses pursuing a practice change, "Sometimes you find the doughnut, and sometimes you find the hole." If you find the doughnut then you have enough strong evidence on which to base your practice. If you find "the hole," then you have a gap in evidence that is ripe for a research project—which begins with formulating a research question, or problem statement. See Figure 4.1.

Developing the Research Question

When the existing literature lacks enough evidence to answer a clinical question, then nurses who have a spirit of inquiry will want to add to the existing body of evidence—and a research study is born! The next step is formulating a research question, also known as a *problem statement*. (For the sake of easier reading, we use the term "research question" as a synonym for "problem statement.") Generally speaking, a *research question* is an interrogative

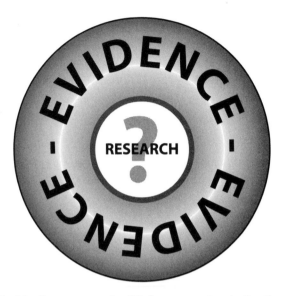

Figure 4.1   The literature search will inform you as to whether there is enough evidence to support a practice change (the doughnut) or there is a need for research (the doughnut hole).

statement that frames a question about the relationship or effect of one variable on another in a specific population. It also is an important factor when selecting an appropriate research design (see Chapters 7 and 12 regarding research designs).

In *quantitative* research, research questions may ask about:

- The characteristics of a specific population (*descriptive* research questions)

- The nature of the relationship between/among variables of interest in a specific population (*correlational* research questions)

- The effect of a variable on another variable or variables in a specific population (*intervention* research questions)

In *qualitative* research, research questions are broader in scope, usually attempting to describe the meaning of a phenomenon to its participants or capture and convey the essence of a phenomenon in a way understandable to others who have not experienced it. Table 4.1 contains examples of these types of research questions.

Table 4.1   Types of Research Questions and Examples

Type of Research Question	Example
Quantitative	
Descriptive	"What is the age distribution, highest nursing degree held, and computer literacy level of inpatient medical-surgical staff nurses?"
Correlational	"Is there a relationship between age and computer literacy level of inpatient medical-nursing staff nurses?"
Intervention	"Is there a difference in computer literacy level in inpatient medical-surgical staff nurses aged 40–60 years who receive online education related to computer use and those who do not?"
Qualitative	
Meaning/Essence	"What is the lived experience of transferring from paper to electronic documentation in inpatient medical-surgical staff nurses?"

There are two components you need to understand further in order to craft good research questions: variables and populations. The following sections describe these components in more detail.

Components of a Research Question: Variables

In order to develop a good research question, you need to understand the concept of variables. Plainly stated, a *variable* is a characteristic that can have more than one value—in other words, the characteristic or property can have several values or categories. Anything that changes and that can be measured can be a research variable. For example, eye color could be considered a variable, as eye color can differ from one person to the next and could be classified into such categories as blue, brown, hazel, green and "other."

In research, the general categories of variables include:

- Independent variables

- Dependent variables

- Extraneous, or confounding, variables

Independent variables. In *experimental* research designs (see Chapter 7 for a detailed discussion of this type of research design), the research question asks if there is a difference between one or more groups of subjects who receive interventions and a group who receives the "standard of care" (or, if ethical, no intervention). The important thing to remember is that, in experimental research designs, the independent variable is the variable: 1) over which the investigator has control, and 2) is assumed to "make the difference" between the two or more groups.

From Table 4.1, consider this research question:

> "Is there a difference in computer literacy level in inpatient medical-surgical staff nurses aged 40–60 years who receive online education related to computer use and those who do not?"

In this study, the investigator has control (one would hope) of the "online education related to computer use," and this form of education is assumed to produce an effect on the nurses' computer literacy. Therefore, the independent variable would be the online education related to computer use (for those of you who are keeping track, this variable does "vary," because the education is either present or it is absent).

In *nonexperimental* research designs, identifying the independent variable can be a bit more elusive. In the case of correlational research questions, the independent variable cannot be manipulated; however, it may occur naturally as first in a sequence or it logically may be assumed that it affects another variable in some way.

 What is an example of a correlational research question?

 What is the relationship between age and incidence of death in adults aged 65–85 years? In this example, the variables of age and death cannot be manipulated, but there may be a strong correlation.

It is important to note that, as Chapter 7 illustrates, correlational designs *cannot* support causality; they simply demonstrate the strength of relationships. For example, in the research question, "Is there a relationship between age and computer literacy level of inpatient medical-nursing staff nurses?" neither the variables of age or of computer literacy are being manipulated. However, one logically could assume that age has an effect on computer literacy, and not the other way around.

Dependent variables. In experimental designs, the dependent variable is contingent upon the independent variable for its effect. Sequentially, the effect on the dependent variable occurs *after* application/occurrence of the independent variable. Consider the following research question:

> "Is there a difference in computer literacy level in inpatient medical-surgical staff nurses aged 40–60 years who receive online education related to computer use and those who do not?"

In this case, the dependent variable is the (hoped for) change in computer literacy in the group receiving the education. In nonexperimental designs, the dependent variable occurs as second (or third, depending on how many dependent variables there are in the study) in a sequence of naturally occurring events, so it may be logically assumed that the preceding variable(s) caused the change.

In the research question, "Is there a relationship between age and computer literacy level of inpatient medical-nursing staff nurses?" there is an unstated assumption that age may have an effect on computer literacy; therefore, computer literacy is the dependent variable.

Extraneous/confounding variables. Although not always identified in the research question, there are always extraneous variables that you need to consider when designing research studies. Extraneous variables are those "other variables" that may affect either the *impact* of the independent variable on the dependent variable (intervention research question) or the *relationship* between the independent and dependent variable (correlational research question). This is often why descriptive research questions are asked.

 What is an example of an intervention research question?

 Will increasing the RN-to-patient staffing ratio from 1:10 to 1:6 affect the incidence of patient falls and pressure ulcers in an elderly inpatient population? In this case, the intervention is the change in RN-to-patient staffing ratio.

For example, here is a descriptive research question:

> "What is the age distribution, highest nursing degree held, and computer literacy level of inpatient medical-surgical staff nurses?"

The results from this study may indicate that the highest level of nursing education may have a mediating or moderating relationship on computer literacy level. In this case, this information would alert an investigator to control for this potential extraneous variable through sample selection (Chapter 8), design of the study (Chapter 7) or by collecting data related to this variable and statistically controlling for it (Chapters 9 and 11).

Once an Independent Variable, Always an Independent Variable?

When first wrestling with the concept of types of variables, it would be easy to assume that once you identify a variable as an independent variable, it will always be an independent variable. Unfortunately, this is not the case. Here's an example that clarifies this.

One of our staff nurses posed the research question, "Is there a relationship between parents' health literacy and their preschool child's body mass index (BMI)?" This is a *correlational* research question in which parental health literacy is the *independent* variable and the child's BMI is the *dependent* variable. Suppose in this study that a strong relationship was found between these two variables, and the staff nurse decides to design an online educational program targeted to improve parents' health literacy (and, hopefully, positively affect children's BMI). A second study might then be proposed with the research question of, "What is the effect of an online health literacy education program on parental health literacy?" Framed as an intervention research question, the health literacy program would be the *independent* variable and parental health literacy would now be the *dependent* variable rather than the *independent* variable, as it was in the first study.

In addition, the child's BMI, which is the *dependent* variable in the first study, might be considered an *extraneous* variable in the second study, as it might be assumed (if a literature search bears this out) that parents of an obese preschooler may be more likely to be attentive to education related to health literacy education, especially when learning to read food labels. Hopefully, it is clear that variables in different research questions can vary (no pun intended) from one type of variable to another.

Defining variables: theoretical and operational definitions. As if identifying the types of variables in a research question is not enough, after you identify variables, you need to define them. There are two definitions to consider:

- **Theoretical/conceptual definition:** This definition of a variable is often called the "encyclopedia" (or, in more current terms the "*Wikipedia*") definition of the variable. This definition is fairly broad and could be described as "defining dictionary terms with other dictionary terms." In other words, the definition is totally "theoretical," and you would not be able to reasonably measure the variable by using this definition.

- **Operational definition:** This definition describes the *exact* method/instrument by which the variable will be measured. It is by this exact definition that another investigator could replicate the variable measurement in the future.

Both definitions are important to consider during the process of selecting the most valid instruments with which to measure the variables of interest, as it is important that the theoretical/conceptual definition and the operational definition are congruent. When incongruence between these two definitions occurs, validity of the measurement of the variable may be in question, and the entire study may be in jeopardy (see Chapter 9 for a discussion of instrument validity).

For example, going back to the set of research questions in Table 4.1, if the theoretical definition of computer literacy is "the ability to successfully complete electronic documentation of the admission, physical assessment, and health history of patients," and the operational definition of computer literacy is "the ability to be able to conduct personal activities such as banking and shopping online," then the theoretical definition of the variable is not in alignment with the operational definition. In this case, an instrument that measures the "ability to successfully complete the steps in an online banking transaction" (which is the operational definition) would not be a valid measurement of the variable "computer literacy of nursing documentation" (which is the theoretical definition). However, in rejected research manuscripts, this type of incongruence has been known to occur.

Q: *After narrowing down a clinical topic, I am having difficulty with developing a research question. Some of my colleagues are saying that what I am interested in can't be measured. Help!*

A: Remember that you need to keep in mind the variable's *operational definition* throughout the development of your research question because you need to be able to measure the variable of interest. Development of conceptual definitions of variables such as *loneliness*, *hope*, or *spirituality* can take a decade or more of work, and the resulting operational definitions and measurement tools can take even longer before they have been validated and the results published. Only a thorough literature search enables you to be certain of whether an appropriate measurement is available or "on the publication horizon."

Components of a Research Question: Populations

Another component of a research question is that of the population to be measured. Although Chapter 8 goes into detail about populations, samples, and sampling techniques, a broad idea of from where or from whom you will collect the data needs to be either stated or implied. For example, the research questions in Table 4.1 state that the data will represent inpatient medical-surgical nurses. When you read about formulating hypotheses in the next section, you'll see that the definition of the population is narrowed down even further.

Research Questions and Feasibility: What Is Going On in the Mind of the Investigator?

As previously mentioned, the research question should guide you in selecting the research design and associated procedures and measurements needed to implement a viable research study. *Feasibility* of the study is a key concept that is kept in mind throughout the development of a research question. The internal dialogue of a nurse scientist who is developing a research question and who is simultaneously concerned about study feasibility might look something like this:

> *Nurse Scientist (NS):* "Okay. My general idea is that I think that I can increase computer literacy in staff nurses by delivering a targeted education program related to the new documentation system, but I need to test this out."
>
> *Evil Twin (ET):* "Well, that's a nice broad statement! What do you mean by computer literacy? Just how will you measure that?"
>
> *NS* [After a literature search]: "I found an article about an online tool that reliably measures accuracy in electronic documentation. So, my conceptual definition will need to state that computer literacy and the ability to document online are similar concepts. My operational definition then would be the measurement of the ability to document online."
>
> *ET:* "Can you get permission to use the tool? How much does it cost? Do you need a dedicated computer to administer the testing? How long does testing take?"
>
> *NS:* "Got it covered. The authors of the instrument made it accessible through the Internet, and all you need to do is register to use it—no cost! It can be administered from any computer with Internet access, and it only takes 10 minutes."
>
> *ET:* "And just who will you convince to go to the trouble of taking this computer literacy test? Do you have access to a population willing to do this?"

NS: "We have 35 medical-surgical units that are 'going live' with electronic documentation within the next four months—I don't think I'll have a problem getting volunteers."

ET: "And what about the educational program? How will it be developed and delivered?"

NS: "Oh, really, ET! You know that I have friends in the Nursing Education Department who would be willing to assist with developing the program. Come to think of it, there are several medical-surgical units that are having difficulty with getting the staff 'onboard' with the electronic documentation. That's where I'll go for this project! In fact, I think that I have a viable research question now—'Is there a difference in computer literacy level in inpatient medical-surgical staff nurses who receive education related to electronic documentation and those who do not?'"

ET: "Next stop, the Institutional Review Board!"

Beyond the Research Question: Determining the Study Purpose

After you finalize the research question and determine it to be feasible, the next step is to develop the purpose of the study, which may also be called the *study aim* or *study objective*. As you can see in the examples in Table 4.2, the study purpose is much broader than the research question, as it describes the wider aspect of what the project should accomplish and also hints, through what verbs are used, at how this might be done.

Table 4.2   Research Questions and Related Study Purposes

Type of Study	Research Question	Purpose/Aims/Objectives
Descriptive	"What is the age distribution, highest nursing degree held, and computer literacy level of inpatient medical-surgical staff nurses?"	The purpose of this study is to *describe* the age distribution, educational levels, and computer literacy of nurses who work on general medical-surgical units.

Type of Study	Research Question	Purpose/Aims/Objectives
Correlational	"Is there a relationship between age and computer literacy level of inpatient medical-surgical staff nurses?"	The aim of this study is to *explore* the relationship between age and computer literacy levels of nurses who work on general medical-surgical units.
Intervention	"Is there a difference in computer literacy level in inpatient medical-surgical staff nurses aged 40–60 years who receive online education related to computer use and those who do not?"	The objective of this study is to *determine* whether online education related to computer use will improve computer literacy in inpatient medical-surgical staff nurses who are 40–60 years of age.
Meaning/ Essence (Phenomenology)	"What is the lived experience of transferring from paper to electronic documentation in inpatient medical-surgical staff nurses?"	The purpose of this study is to *explicate* the lived experience of inpatient medical-surgical staff nurses who transfer from paper to electronic patient documentation.

Q: *Is it necessary to know what kind of study you are conducting in order to write the research question, or does the research question determine the type of study being conducted?*

A: The research question is one of the key drivers of the resultant research design; however, it is not the only factor. Ethical considerations and feasibility (e.g., access to a subject population and resources) also are considerations.

For example, the words *describe, explore,* and *explicate* in a study purpose statement denote that the research topic is probably not well defined in the existing literature, and preliminary exploration of the topic needs to be performed. In these cases, descriptive or correlational study designs (with their accompanying methodologies and procedures) are appropriate. In the case of *determining* whether an intervention will make a difference in an outcome, an experimental design would most likely be used.

Beyond the Research Question: Formulating Research Hypotheses

When you finalize the research question and study purpose, the last step in this phase of the process is to determine whether you can propose research hypotheses. But first, a definition is in order—a *research hypothesis* is a declarative statement that indicates a relationship between two or more variables and suggests an answer to the related research question. Moreover, it also indicates the population that is to be studied. Table 4.3 contains research hypotheses that might be formulated for some of the earlier research questions.

Table 4.3   Research Questions and Potential Research Hypotheses

Type of Study	Research Question	Potential Research Hypothesis
Descriptive	"What is the age distribution, highest nursing degree held and computer literacy level of inpatient medical-surgical staff nurses?"	There will be significant differences in computer literacy scores (DV) according to age (IV) and highest nursing degree (IV) attained in inpatient medical-surgical staff nurses employed in a multicampus hospital system.
Correlational	"Is there a relationship between age and computer literacy level of inpatient medical-nursing staff nurses?"	There will be an inverse relationship between computer literacy (DV) and age (IV) in inpatient medical-surgical staff nurses employed in a multicampus hospital system.
Intervention	"Is there a difference in computer literacy level in inpatient medical-surgical staff nurses aged 40–60 years who receive online education related to computer use and those who do not?"	Medical-surgical staff nurses aged 40–60 years who are employed in a multicampus hospital system who receive an online education module related to computer use (IV) will score higher in a test of computer literacy (DV) than those nurses who do not receive the educational module.

Abbreviations: *IV = Independent Variable*
DV = Dependent Variable

The "Educated Guess": The Research Hypothesis

It could be said that the hypothesis is an "educated guess" of what the relationship between/ among variables will be after data are statistically analyzed and interpreted. To maintain scientific honesty, hypotheses are always formulated at the beginning of the study (no fair peeking at the data first!). Additionally, the term "educated guess" comes from the fact that the relationships that hypotheses state should be based on either previous research and/or from the relationships posited in theoretical frameworks.

For example, if findings from previous studies have suggested that online education has been useful as a teaching method for staff nurse education, then it would be reasonable to formulate the research hypothesis, "Medical-surgical staff nurses employed in a multicampus hospital system who receive an online education module related to computer use will score higher in a test of computer literacy than those nurses who do not receive the educational module."

However, if there was no existing research evidence or theoretical framework on which to base the hunch that online education is useful in providing staff nurse education, then the research hypothesis might be, "There will be a difference between computer literacy test scores of medical-surgical staff nurses employed in a multicampus hospital system who receive an online education module related to computer use and those who do not." There will be more discussion about these two types of research hypotheses shortly.

The Dreaded "Null Hypothesis"

Lurking in the background behind the educated guess of the research hypothesis is the specter of the "null hypothesis" (also known as the *statistical hypothesis*). This hypothesis is simpler to develop, as it *always* states that there is *no relationship between/among variables*, including finding *differences* between/among groups of subjects.

For example, the null hypothesis related to the research hypotheses stated previously would be, "There will be *no* difference between computer literacy scores of nurses who receive online education related to computer use and those who do not." As discussed in Chapter 11, if a statistical significance is found, then the null hypothesis can be rejected. However, that does *not* automatically mean that the research hypothesis is supported—this is due to the possible ways in which research hypotheses can be stated.

Q: *I can't wait until Chapter 11 on statistics—in a nutshell, what does "statistical significance" mean?*

A: Statistical significance (expressed as a probability, or *p* value) is the probability that the results of an intervention (or, in the case of a correlational study, a relationship) occurred purely by chance. For example, if you see a result reported as "p = .04", this denotes that the possibility of the results occurring purely by chance is 4%. In research, one is never 100% sure of anything; however, as a research consumer, you need to evaluate whether a 4% *possibility* of the intervention not working is acceptable or not. For example, in the use of some very toxic or very expensive drugs, you might want to see that chance decrease to 1% (or even less). But that's a discussion for Chapter 11.

Further Characteristics of Hypotheses: Directional Versus Nondirectional Hypotheses

The reason that rejecting a null hypothesis does not automatically support the research hypothesis can be demonstrated by referring to our two earlier research hypotheses. At first glance, the difference between the two is minor; however, using a directional (one-tailed) versus a nondirectional (two-tailed) hypothesis has implications for statistical analysis and interpretation of the findings. Let's investigate the difference between these two research hypotheses a bit further from a nonstatistical point of view.

Directional hypotheses. First, let's examine research hypothesis #1:

Staff nurses who receive an online education module related to computer use will score higher in a test of computer literacy than those nurses who do not receive the educational module.

This hypothesis identifies a direction to look for in the data that is collected; specifically, you would expect to see *higher* computer literacy scores in the nurses receiving the online education. This type of hypothesis is known as a *directional* (or *one-tailed*) *hypothesis* because it specifies the direction in which you would look for the difference or the variable relationship.

So, if the data indicate that the nurses receiving the education scored significantly higher than those who did not, you could reject the null hypothesis and accept the research hypothesis. However, what would happen if the nurses who did *not* receive the online education actually scored significantly *higher* than those who received it? Would the null hypothesis be rejected? Yes. Would the research hypothesis be supported? No—because the direction in which the "difference" was predicted was not found (ouch!). Fortunately, as most (good) research hypotheses are grounded in past research evidence or theory, this rarely happens.

Nondirectional hypotheses. Now, consider research hypothesis #2:

> There will be a difference between computer literacy test scores of medical-surgical staff nurses employed in a multicampus hospital system who receive an online education module related to computer use and those who do not.

In this hypothesis, there is no specific direction stated; the hypothesis simply states that there will be a difference/relationship between variables. In this case, if the null hypothesis is rejected, would the research hypothesis be supported? Yes, because the way in which the research hypothesis was stated means that it does not matter in which direction the difference was found, as long as one was found (Actually, it does not matter to the statistical test, but it may matter to the investigator).

Try It Now!

The purpose of this exercise is to encourage you to develop multiple types of research questions from one clinical issue. The ability to do this increases the chances of success in developing a viable research study.

Scenario: You are a staff nurse on a surgical cardiac step-down unit where patients commonly have chest tubes removed. You think that these patients typically are very anxious about this procedure, and you decide to do something to decrease their anxiety (and possibly increase their satisfaction with their hospital experience). Using the following table, develop a research question that would fit each category, and then develop related study purposes and hypotheses (where appropriate). *Hint: This table would be appropriate for a multitude of other clinical issues, so feel free to substitute your own.*

Category of Research Question	My Research Question Is...	The Purpose of the Study Would Be...	Possible Hypotheses Would Be...
Descriptive			
Correlational			
Intervention			
Meaning/ Essence			

References

Benner, P. (1984). *Novice to expert: Excellence and power in clinical nursing practice.* Upper Saddle River, NJ: Prentice Hall.

Huang, X., Lin, J., & Demner-Fushman, D. (2006). Evaluation of PICO as a knowledge representation for clinical questions. *American Medical Informatics Association Annual Symposium Proceedings*, 359–363.

Schardt, C., Adams, M. B., Owens, T., Keitz, S., & Fontelo, P. (2007). Utilization of the PICO framework to improve searching PubMed for clinical questions. *Medical Informatics and Decision Making*, 7:16. doi:10.1186/1472-6947-7-16. Retrieved from http://www.biomedcentral.com/1472-6947/7/16

Straus, S. E., Glasziou, P., Richardson, W. S., & Haynes, R. B. (2011). *Evidence-based medicine: How to practice and teach it,* (4th ed.). London: Churchill Livingstone: Elsevier.

"None of us is as smart as all of us."

–Ken Blanchard

Forming Research Teams

5

Kathleen Russell-Babin

You wouldn't think of caring for a chronic obstructive pulmonary disease (COPD) patient without the collaboration of a physician, a respiratory therapist, a pharmacist, and sometimes a physical therapist. The relative strengths of each discipline are needed in order to meet the patient's needs and secure the best outcomes. The stronger the collaboration and teamwork, the better the patient outcomes. The same is true for completing a research study. A carefully selected team of a variety of health professions with the right characteristics ensures the best outcome. This chapter describes the composition of a multidisciplinary research team and how to ensure an effectively functioning research team.

Team Composition

Your research team will have to meet the challenges of selecting the strongest research design possible for the circumstances, develop an acceptable data analysis plan, prepare a proposal to accompany the Institutional Review Board (IRB) application, and create communication vehicles for the results of the research, which may include but are not limited to scholarly journal articles. To put together a successful research team, you need to consider the following:

WHAT YOU'LL LEARN IN THIS CHAPTER

- In order to develop a strong research team, you need to consider multiple foundational characteristics.

- A variety of research-specific and general leadership abilities will be needed to ensure progress.

- Ways to maximize team effectiveness and productivity are available and should be utilized.

- How to build off your own strengths and weaknesses

- Socio-political-economic factors

- Size of the team

These items are described in more detail in the following sections.

Building Off Your Own Strengths and Weaknesses

The first thing you should do when putting together your team is ask yourself: What strengths do I need to have in formulating the team to accomplish these objectives? The initial decision on team composition rests upon a careful examination of your own strengths and weaknesses. Consider the following questions:

- How knowledgeable am I in selecting the strongest research design possible for the situation?

- If the study is quantitative, do I understand the strengths and limitations of the research method involved? Do I have the statistics background in order to select appropriate statistical tools to analyze the data?

- If the study is qualitative, do I understand the various qualitative design options? Do I have experience in theme and category analysis? Do I have experience in using a software program or analysis process that will produce credible results?

- How strong are my writing skills? Have I had sufficient experience in scholarly writing to be able to share my results broadly in the nursing community?

The results of the preceding self-assessment will direct you to search for people who can fill in the skill gaps you may have in the formulation of your research study. Answering all these points will ensure you have the technical research skills on board for a successful study. This is only the first of the factors to consider in team composition.

Taking Socio-Political-Economic Factors Into Consideration

A second level of consideration is the socio-political-economic one. Who are your key stakeholders in this research? Your study will need financial and other organizational support from key individuals inside and outside of your organization.

Ask yourself: How do I know who I should add to my team to strengthen the research plan's acceptability to key stakeholders? Consider the following questions to learn the answer to this question:

- If my study is being funded, what expertise might outside funders expect?

- Does the financial or sociopolitical support rely upon on my team having a team member with a doctorate degree?

- Do I need to include key influential leaders as members of the team?

- Do I need to include someone who is representative of the study participants involved in planning the research study?

The last question posed in the preceding list is becoming an increasingly important one in research circles in health care. The federal government is sponsoring patient-centered research as a means to improving patient outcomes (www.pcori.org). Interest is particularly high on learning more about improving patients' participation in their own health care decisions and in how they may partner to improve their health. To that end, the studies' approvals are prioritized based on such objectives. Members of the intended population are expected to be active members of the research team.

Q: *Who is an example of someone of influence whom I would need to help move my study along?*

A: Perhaps your manager or director would be helpful to you in navigating any administrative approvals in the environment of your study. Another example would be if your study is about medication management, perhaps a Pharm. D. would be a helpful member of your team.

Determining the Size of the Team

The next logical question is how big should this team be? No hard-and-fast rules exist for the answer to this question. McCann (2007) noted that teams of more than 8 members may not be the most productive. Did you ever wonder how the contributions of scholarly articles with 10 authors were managed? It seems highly likely that their contributions varied tremendously in scope and amount. Depending upon your sociopolitical content, 4 or 5 team members, including yourself, are the maximum that are really needed.

Finding your Team Members

A fundamental consideration in finding team members is to assure that individuals involved have and will devote their time to the research. You need to give them at least a general sense of what you expect of them so they can judge their capacity to provide it. Very often in novice research studies, minimal to no compensation is available for their time. Can they accommodate the voluntary nature of your request?

The next basic consideration in selecting team members has to do with their expertise. Sometimes you need people with very specific expertise. For example, do you need someone who has previously done health literacy research and is highly knowledgeable in it?

What are some available sources of team members you might access who may be able to assist you? Is there a nursing research department or a division of the nursing education department devoted to research? Do you know any local nursing leaders who have performed a research study at work or in their program of study? They might be enthusiastic mentors.

Q: *We do not have a nurse researcher/scientist or a statistician in our institution. What should we do?*

A: Bettger and Granger (2012) suggested that researchers explore whether schools of nursing affiliated with your organization have or would be willing to develop a research partnership. Schools of nursing have many more doctorally prepared nurses than many practice arenas. If a statistician is still needed, is there someone in performance improvement or other departments with these skills who may help you? If not, many statisticians perform independent contractor work and can provide invaluable service.

Role of the Research Team Leader

Although you may have a number of highly skilled individuals on your team, the study will not likely progress smoothly without leadership. The study team leader is usually the principal investigator (PI). This is the person who is assuming full responsibility for all aspects of the study and who usually has the vision for what the study is to accomplish. Some of the most important roles the study team leader must fulfill include:

- Communicating the vision for the study to the team and any stakeholders

- Assuming final responsibility for the IRB application, including the study proposal

- Monitoring study protocols and progress, assuring compliance to human subject protection concerns, and faithfulness to the study plan

- Interim study communication among the team and to stakeholders

- Team analysis of findings

- Reporting of final analyses

In addition to several roles that you'll need to fill, you have several tasks you'll need to perform.

Common Tasks

As the leader of a research team, you will have many duties in addition to coordinating the research study. Some of the most common tasks include:

- **Manage timelines.** Deadlines exist for nursing department approvals, IRB applications, for grants (if applied for), and sometimes for internal goal achievement.

- **Develop a communication plan.** As the leader, you must ensure an active communication plan is developed. Timely communication to stakeholders is very important, whether that involves a steering committee in more complicated studies or one-on-one communications with key people.

- **Keep the team abreast of current developments.** The research team must all be aligned with the most recent developments at all times.

  For example, in a medication reconciliation study, clinical pharmacists, staff nurses, and a nurse researcher teamed to investigate the effectiveness of having a pharmacist at the bedside on improving the accuracy of medication reconciliation. Ongoing communication about practical aspects of the study was required in order to make sure the project went smoothly. Such things as laptop access, data worksheet collection, and space availability for the bedside pharmacist on the unit were addressed through regular communication.

- **Hold team meetings.** Team meetings may need to be held, whether they are in person or electronic. Many hospitals have support for conference calls. Check with your organization to see if they participate in a conference-call service. Sometimes it is possible to simply use concise and meaningful email exchanges in order to accomplish the intent of a meeting.

- **Harness the talents of team members.** The leader needs to plan how to leverage the talents of the research team to create the best product possible. Using the strengths of individuals involved instead of pushing everyone to excel in all facets of the study will produce a greater working team. For example, one member may be more experienced in IRB policies, whereas another may be stronger on the pros and cons of various research designs. Use that knowledge to strengthen your team.

As you can see, a team leader has many responsibilities. But a leader must also possess some important leadership characteristics in order to effectively lead the team through its paces.

Characteristics of a Good Leader

The research team leader is not just the principal investigator or the senior research official. As the team leader, you are the team member who participates in and maximizes teamwork, and at the same time you are usually the originator of the idea and developer of the proposal. To accomplish this, you must have a strong vision of the research intent. Clear communications must convey expectations with timely constructive feedback to members on progress.

Q: *I thought the person who came up with the research idea would be the team leader, but this sounds like it's not always the case. When would the team leader be someone other than the idea originator?*

A: Sometimes a novice researcher may have a great idea, but may not have the skills to lead a team in planning and implementing a study. In this case, the experienced researcher may be the team leader and can mentor the novice researcher.

Also, as the leader you should encourage team members to share their perspectives and to teach and guide each other in their areas of strength. For example, several pros and cons will be identified in the search for the most optimal research design. All team members must challenge each other with alternatives in order to ultimately reach consensus on the best design.

The team leader needs organizational skills in order to meet timelines and objectives. You, as the team leader, can best prepare to organize the study by having a thorough understanding of all IRB application and funding source requirements (or working with a mentor who has that knowledge).

The team leader must celebrate each milestone success, large or small, with the team. Celebrate achieving IRB approval and obtaining a satisfactory sample! This is especially important because it is very rare for the team to have any form of compensation for their efforts. Choosing motivated and interested parties and celebrating with them as a team is what works.

Planning to Maximize Team Productivity

Careful examination of expectations from the outset helps to keep the team focused and productive. Is the answer to the research question needed before the next organizational budget cycle or formal goal-setting process? This will help set the timeline for the study. For example, if a staff nurse is conducting pilot research on medication administration interruptions, it would be optimal that the results be completed and findings communicated before the organizational goals are set for the following fiscal year if the study has the potential to be spread more widely throughout the organization in the future.

At the beginning of the study, you should itemize all steps in the journey of a research study with their associated timeline and responsible parties to help everyone stay on track throughout what can be a long process. The team leader, with input from team members, should generate a table that includes all tasks, no matter how insignificant (see Figure 5.1). An important area to include on the list is the timeline for reporting outside the research team. Formal and informal agreements that formulated your financial and organizational approvals may govern these reporting timelines. Overall, this tool serves as both the to-do list for everyone and as the performance checklist. The resulting tool can be part of the ongoing agenda of team meetings. It can also be used as part of a status-reporting tool to organizational administrators.

The team needs to have a clear understanding of the hurdles they must overcome on the road to front-end study approval. Getting the required protection of human subjects training completed is an early task to complete. Some organizations require that nursing research studies be approved by a body of their peers, or a scientific review committee such as a nursing research committee, before it moves to IRB approval. Many times, it is fruitful to have an informal meeting with the IRB personnel before documents submission. This often sheds new light on the requirements associated with the specific research plan. Both of these processes can act as consultative steps in developing your final research plan and IRB application (see Chapter 14 for more information about IRB approval).

Element	Responsible Party	Due Date/Status Completion
Complete human subjects training	S. Smith, RN M. Jones, RN L. Biostats, MS	November–December
Refine research target	Research team	December 1
Get stakeholder feedback on target and related concepts	S. Smith, RN	December 15
Compare and contrast various research designs	Research team	December 31
Assess sample size needed	L. Biostats, MS	December 31
Draft proposal	S. Smith, RN	January 31
Finalize proposal and processes	S. Smith, RN M. Jones, RN L. Biostats, MS S. Smith, RN	February 15 January 31
Complete nursing research committee requirements and present at next available meeting	S. Smith, RN M. Jones, RN	March 15
Complete IRB application	M. Jones, RN	March 31
Celebrate IRB approval	Research team	May 15
Schedule monthly meetings to discuss progress and challenges	S. Smith, RN	Beginning May 15
Prepare copies of study tools and materials	M. Jones, RN	May 15
Establish firm study start point	S. Smith, RN M. Jones, RN	May 15
Ensure intra-rater consistency in research data collection processes by practicing data collection and comparing results	S. Smith, RN M. Jones, RN	April 30
Prepare timelines for intervention(s)	S. Smith, RN M. Jones, RN	April 30
Communicate plans to relevant stakeholders	S. Smith, RN	May 1
Celebrate data collection completion	Research team	August 30
Data analysis	L. Biostats, MS	September 30
Data review and conclusions	Research team	October 31

Figure 5.1   Sample to-do list for a research study for S. Smith, RN, Principal Investigator

Just as two minds can improve upon the ideas of one, sharing the research plan with a broader steering committee is sometimes helpful in studies that have broad impact. Inviting feedback on your plan early in the development process is best. This helps identify forces that may impede your study; it can also enhance your study by identifying issues of which you might otherwise have been unaware. Further, it invites constructive criticism that a research team may not develop as they become enamored with their own ideas. This produces a stronger plan in the end, although the feedback may not always be what you want to hear.

Pulling It All Together

A staff nurse wanted to investigate whether cough and deep breathe or incentive spirometry was the appropriate therapy postoperatively to prevent pulmonary complications in abdominal and chest trauma patients on a medical-surgical unit. An evidence review was completed with a team that included a nurse scientist, a statistician, a respiratory therapist, and staff nurses. Members of the trauma medical team/advanced practice nurses (APNs) were invited but were unable to attend. The team reviewed the evidence for several weeks. The completed review (Rupp, Miley, & Russell-Babin, 2013) found that both cough and deep breathe and incentive spirometry were equally effective.

When the results were shared with the trauma medical team/APNs, the findings were questioned. This was not entirely unexpected as the trauma medical team/APNs were not part of the working team from the beginning. What was not expected was that a request was made that a research study be developed to test the use of a visual prompt for cough and deep breathe and compare the outcomes of those patients to patients using incentive spirometers. It turned out that the medical team/APNs group did not doubt the mechanisms of treatment so much as the adherence to treatment. They believed the incentive spirometer represented a visual cue to act. The bad news was that more work was required to move down the path of translation of evidence. The good news was that input into the plan was broadened by appropriate stakeholders.

So who comprised the new research team? The staff nurse for the original evidence review became the principal investigator (PI) and team leader. The nurse scientist and statistician supported him with the research design plan. The trauma APN and lead physician joined the research team for clinical input and stakeholder representation. A nurse educator was included on the team as the intervention would rely heavily on staff and patient education. The staff nurse PI informally brought his nurse manager into the team in order to pave the way for all activity to come. No external funding or stakeholders existed beyond this. The end result was a complementary group of professionals highly invested in making the research study a success.

The staff nurse PI met with each of the parties involved before crafting the research plan for the IRB application. He kept his nurse manager in the loop at all times so she would support his scheduling needs and communication requirements to the nurses on the postoperative unit. He shared his draft with his team and got their feedback early on. He prepared for the nursing research committee and attended the meeting to obtain approval. He made modifications to the plan based on their feedback, communicated these changes to his research team, and submitted the final plan to IRB. Due to all the preparation, the IRB granted approval for the research plan. Virtual celebration ensued!

The team formulated their table of actions and timelines in order to ensure the study would move forward. This, too, was communicated with unit leadership. The staff nurse PI secured a regular update on the trauma team's scheduled meetings.

Roles of Team Members

In a research study, you may not always be the team leader; you may be a team member and that is an important role! You've been invited to be a team member because you possess skills that are important to the success of the study. But keep in mind that team members should have sufficient time to devote to the study, need to be timely in their responses to requests from the team leaders, and meet the expected timelines. In addition, team members need to provide helpful, constructive feedback.

Try It Now!

Think of a potential topic you are considering for a research study. Now formulate your research "dream team"! Did you consider all stakeholders? Who would be the Principal Investigator/Team Leader? What special knowledge and skills would each member contribute to the success of your study?

References

Bettger, J. P., & Granger, B. B. (2012). Engaging research partners to advance clinical inquiry. *AACN Advanced Critical Care, 23*(4), 471–478.

McCann, M. (2007). The challenges encountered during a collaborative research project. *Journal of Renal Care, 33*(3), 139–142.

Rupp, M., Miley, H., & Russell-Babin, K. (2013). Incentive spirometry in postoperative abdominal/thoracic surgery patients. *AACN Advanced Critical Care, 24*(3), 255–263.

"The librarian isn't a clerk who happens to work at a library. A librarian is a data hound, a guide, a sherpa and a teacher. The librarian is the interface between reams of data and the untrained but motivated user."

–Seth Godin

Conducting a Literature Search and Review

Catherine M. Boss
Barbara Williams

Suppose you are a novice nurse caring for a diabetic patient who is prescribed a number of medications with which you are not familiar. You want to look up the medications but want to also make sure that you get the most up-to-date, accurate, and comprehensive information. You then seek out an expert, the nurse practitioner on your unit/service, who assists you in locating the most definitive sources to obtain the information you need so that you don't waste time using less reliable sources. The nurse practitioner remains available to answer any questions you may have about the medications and the care of your patient. After you have obtained the information and have clarified your questions with the nurse practitioner, you are better able to assess the patient and make decisions about the care you give. In the same way, the librarian is the expert who can assist in locating the most comprehensive evidence for your literature review. You can then go on to evaluate and organize the literature with the guidance of an experienced nurse researcher as needed. In this chapter, you will learn how to conduct a literature search, how to organize and evaluate the studies retrieved, and how to write the literature review section of your proposal.

6

WHAT YOU'LL LEARN IN THIS CHAPTER

- A literature review is conducted to answer a clinical question or to explore a research question.

- A multiple database literature search is needed to locate relevant research evidence.

- Specific search strategies will organize your search and make it more thorough.

- Strategies exist that will help you to organize the literature you have retrieved and to write your literature review.

The Literature Review

The purpose of a *literature review* is to orient the reader to what is known and not known about the topic of interest. You should always start with a question about the topic and then gather the literature, appraise the studies, and interpret the findings. The review should be unbiased, meaning that you don't exclude studies when the results are different from what you expected or different from what you prefer. The review should also be thorough and up to date (Polit & Beck, 2010). However, we are getting a bit ahead of ourselves. Prior to conducting the review, it is necessary to know how to first find the literature that is relevant to your question.

The First Step: Meeting Your Medical Librarian

If you have attempted to conduct a search on your own and have not found any results or have only found studies with negative results, you may have reached an impasse. Searching the literature for evidence can present challenges for a busy nurse due to the sheer volume of literature available. How do you find relevant research-based evidence amidst the volumes and volumes of irrelevant literature? Meet the medical librarian, a specialist in searching the literature who is able to find the best, most authoritative, and relevant medical evidence—in a sense, the ultimate search engine. You can either collaborate with a librarian for different search terms and search strategies or request a librarian-mediated literature search. Either of these options can help to locate relevant research studies in a shorter amount of time.

Q: *Why would I go to a medical librarian to locate evidence when so much material is available online?*

A: When you have a medical issue beyond your expertise, you generally seek the advice of a specialist. So why not do the same when it comes to searching the literature by seeking the advice of a librarian or by scheduling a training session? As an untrained searcher, the haphazard nature of finding evidence can lead you to results of questionable quality. Also, not all literature is available online, and the literature you miss may be vital to your review. Read on for a comprehensive explanation of why and how librarians can be helpful.

Librarians understand a variety of search engines and interfaces and have the ability to locate resources beyond the electronically published literature, particularly the older published literature, unpublished literature, and grey literature publications. (Grey literature publications are publications that are unconventional, fugitive, and sometimes ephemeral, such as fact sheets, technical reports, white papers, statistical reports, market research, workshop summaries, and dissertations; they are freely accessible through the Internet.) Medical librarians are uniquely qualified to teach you how to find evidence-based, discipline-specific information in the journal literature. A training session between you and a medical librarian provides a collaboration that combines the clinician's subject knowledge with the librarian's searching skills, yielding the best results.

Locating Evidence

There is no ideal database (i.e., organized collection of journal articles, book chapters, or images) for "one-stop shopping" when doing a comprehensive literature search for evidence. Each database uses different vocabularies to organize its content. When you look in more than one database, you will find more relevant evidence such as research studies. See Table 6.1 for a list of databases and their URLs.

Table 6.1   Useful Research Evidence Databases

Database	Free or License	URL
CINAHL	License	www.ebscohost.com/nursing
PubMed	Free	http://pubmed.gov
Cochrane Database of Systematic Reviews	License	www.thecochranelibrary.com
TRIP	Free	www.tripdatabase.com
Google Scholar	Free	http://scholar.google.com/

Q: *Is there a difference in the quality of content I get, depending on whether I use subscription-based databases versus using a free service or Google Scholar for my research evidence?*

A: Yes there is a difference in what is retrieved from a licensed product, a free service, or Google Scholar. Each database uses its own terminology, taxonomy, system interfaces, and logic to include articles in its database. Also, the content varies from database to database. These differences affect the words a nurse would use to find relevant articles. For example, dissertation abstracts or an original research article from the 1940s may be retrieved in one database but not another.

The following sections include a description of the databases outlined in Table 6.1.

Cumulative Index to Nursing and Allied Health Literature

The Cumulative Index to Nursing and Allied Health Literature (CINAHL) provides indexing of the nursing, biomedicine, health sciences librarianship, alternative/complementary medicine, consumer health, and allied health literature, as well as publications from the National League for Nursing, the American Nurses' Association, and the Cochrane Collaboration. In addition, CINAHL provides access to dissertations, selected conference proceedings, standards of practice, audiovisuals, book chapters, legal cases, clinical innovations, critical paths, research instruments, and clinical trials.

PubMed

Another key source of evidence is PubMed, the United States National Library of Medicine's database of biomedical journal literature. Free access to this database became available in 1997 when Vice President Al Gore supported free access by Americans to medical literature to be consistent with President Clinton's government initiative to improve the quality of health care in the United States. PubMed now has more than 23 million citations from more than 5,600 journals in the biomedical literature from 1946 to the present. The database includes references that have been published electronically ahead of print, as well as publisher-supplied citations that may not be biomedical in nature.

Cochrane Database of Systematic Reviews

The Cochrane Collaboration is an international, independent, not-for-profit organization of more than 31,000 contributors from more than 120 countries. The contributors work together to produce systematic reviews of health care interventions, known as Cochrane Reviews, intended to help providers, practitioners, and patients make informed decisions about health care. The Cochrane Database of Systematic Reviews is the most comprehensive, reliable, and relevant source of evidence on which to base these decisions.

Turning Research Into Practice

Another free database is the Turning Research into Practice (TRIP) database. The TRIP has been online since 1997, when it was first published as an Excel spreadsheet. It was designed to help rapidly answer clinical questions. The idea was to bring together all the "evidence-based" content in one searchable place. The TRIP has filters on the right side of the page to make it easier for clinicians to find the most suitable content. Publishers are classified based on their output or research results. By clicking a particular type of evidence, a clinician can restrict research results to just those types of articles.

The Joanna Briggs Institute

The Joanna Briggs Institute (JBI) is a not-for-profit research and development organization based at the University of Adelaide in South Australia. The Institute collaborates internationally with more than 70 entities across the world to promote and support the synthesis, transfer, and utilization of evidence through identifying feasible, appropriate, meaningful, and effective health care practices to assist in the improvement of health care outcomes globally. The Institute and its collaborators produce a comprehensive range of resources across seven publication types: Evidence-Based Recommended Practices, Evidence Summaries, Best Practice Information Sheets, Systematic Reviews, Consumer Information Sheets, Systematic Review Protocols, and Technical Reports.

Google Scholar

Google Scholar, which is also free, provides a simple way to broadly search for scholarly literature. From Google Scholar, the clinician can search across many disciplines and sources: articles, theses, books, abstracts, and court opinions from academic publishers, professional societies, online repositories, universities, and other websites in the world of scholarly research. Google Scholar ranks documents by weighing the full text of each document, where it was published, and who it was written by, as well as how often and how recently it has been cited in other scholarly literature.

 Are some databases better than others for certain research topics?

 This depends on the topic and the discipline. For example, CINAHL is the largest and most comprehensive database for nursing and allied health and so would be better for searching topics of interest to nursing. PubMed's content is primarily medical (but includes nursing and allied health) and so would be better for searching topics of a biomedical nature.

Identifying a Research Article

Findings from previous studies are the most important type of literature to include in a review (Polit & Beck, 2010). However, a novice researcher may not always understand how to distinguish a research article from other types of literature. A research article that describes a study and is written by the researcher(s) who conducted the study is known as a *primary source*. This kind of study may vary (e.g., experiment, survey, interview, etc.), but in all cases the raw data was collected and analyzed by the authors, and the conclusions were drawn from the results of that analysis. Scientists and scholars publish research articles to disseminate the results of their work, and they are nearly always published in a peer-reviewed journal.

A *secondary source* is a description of a study, or studies, that is written by someone other than the researcher(s) who conducted the study (Polit & Beck, 2010). For example, a review article provides a great overview of the existing literature on a topic and can suggest new research direction, strengthen support for existing theories, or identify patterns among existing research studies (Coulter, 2012).

> **Q:** *When I'm searching a topic, should the majority of my articles be primary sources?*
>
> **A:** The majority of the articles should be primary sources. Secondary sources do not contain as much detail as primary sources, and you may miss critical information. Furthermore, secondary sources may not be objective (Polit & Beck, 2010).

One can identify a research article because it generally includes the following components:

- **The abstract:** This is a brief description at the beginning of the article that summarizes the study.

- **Introduction:** The introduction demonstrates that the authors are aware of existing studies and/or theories and are planning to contribute to the existing body of knowledge in a meaningful way. This section includes the following elements, but the headings can vary depending on the requirements of the journal to which the article is submitted:

  - The theoretical framework, if there is one

  - The major variables (phenomena) in the study

- The research purpose, question/hypothesis

- A review of the existing literature on the topic

- The significance of and need for the study

- **Methods:** This section describes how the research was conducted and can be quite detailed to allow other researchers the ability to verify or replicate the methods used in the study. It includes:

  - The study design

  - The sample and sampling plan

  - How the data were collected and analyzed

- **Results:** This section describes the outcome of the data analysis. It typically includes charts, graphics, and tables that portray the results of the study.

- **Discussion:** This section describes:

  - The author's interpretation of the results

  - How the findings compare to previous studies

  - Implications of the results of the study for practice

- **References:** All research articles include a reference list of those books, articles, and other source material that were cited in the article.

Conducting a Literature Search

When starting your literature search for the evidence, you should follow the steps described earlier in the book. Begin with a clinical question (Chapter 3) and then develop a PICOT question (Chapters 2 and 4). If insufficient evidence is found to support a change in practice and a research study is warranted, then you'll develop a research question or hypothesis for a study (Chapter 4).

Next, you identify the key concepts of the question and make a list of those key concepts. The most successful searches of the journal literature focus on two to four key concepts. For example, to find evidence on the question of whether eating chocolate can have positive health effects on middle-aged women, the primary key concept would be "chocolate." "Health effects", "middle-age", and "women" are secondary concepts of interest.

The next step is to select a database to search. Begin the search by typing into the query box only the key concept—not the entire PICOT question. This is called *natural language searching*. Use the other concepts from your list to add additional terms to your search and to limit or filter the number of references found.

Let's walk through a quick example using CINAHL:

1. Locate the *Advanced Search* link just beneath the query box. Enter the key concept in the first query box (see Figure 6.1).

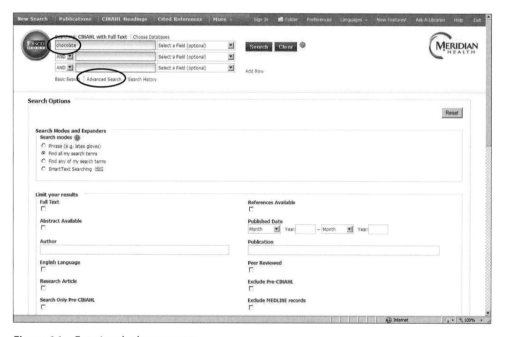

Figure 6.1   Entering the key concept

2. Scroll down the page to select limits appropriate for the question, such as publication years, inpatients, language, and human studies. In the case of the chocolate search, use the *age groups* and *gender* limits to retrieve results on middle-aged females (see Figure 6.2).

3. There is also a limit box for *publication type* (see Figure 6.3).

4. Check as many limits as needed.

5. If the resulting references listed are not relevant, deselect some of the limits and search again.

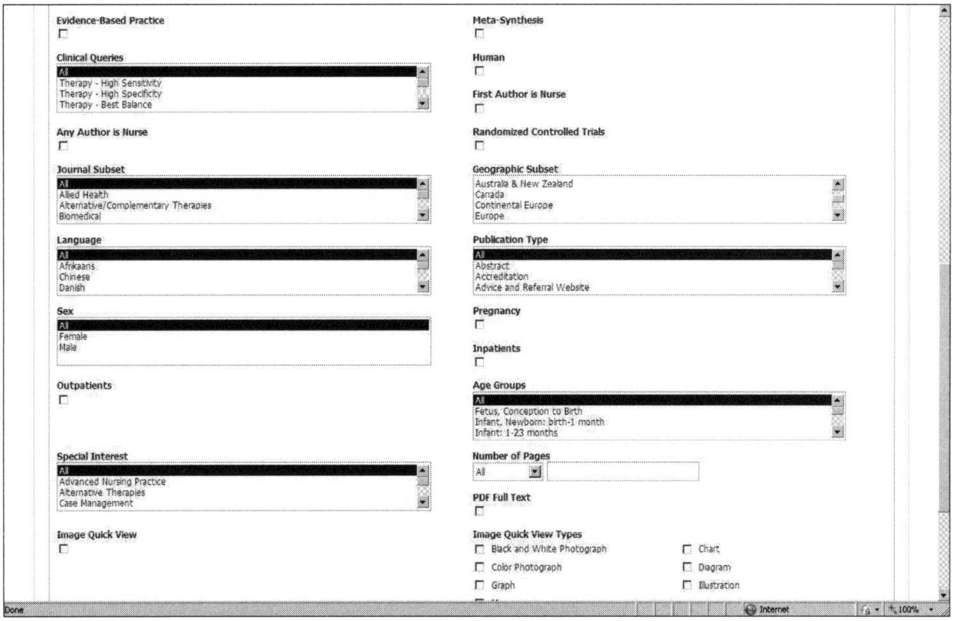

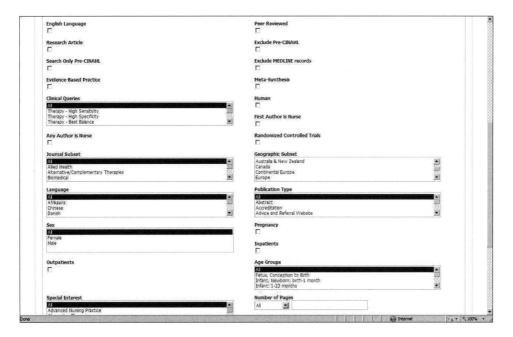

Figure 6.2   Limiting the search

Figure 6.3   Publication type

To find research articles in CINAHL that cover or compare the key concept and a second concept, use the advanced search mode to enter the second concept into a second query box. Choose the Boolean operators AND, OR, or NOT found at the beginning or end of the query box to combine the two ideas (see Figure 6.1). Here's a quick description of how to use these operators:

- **AND:** Narrows a search, locating articles that cover *both* concepts

- **OR:** Broadens a search to include *all* articles about each concept

- **NOT:** Eliminates a concept entered in a query box

For example, when searching for the health effects of chocolate in middle-aged women who are not diabetic, enter the concept of "diabetes" in the third query box and use the NOT operator to eliminate articles related to diabetes from the results.

Now let's consider a search with PubMed:

PubMed uses filters, located on the left side of the query page, to limit a search query. Again, check as many filters as needed and deselect a filter if the results are not relevant. If animal study research is not needed, for example, select the *human* filter. If articles written in a foreign language are not needed, Show Additional Filters, select Languages, and select English.

To cover or compare the key concept chocolate with the second concept health effects, connect the two concepts using a Boolean operator typed in all caps. For example, type "chocolate AND health effects" in the search query box to find research articles on the health effects of chocolate.

Sorting and Evaluating the Results

When you are unable to locate sufficient evidence to support a practice change, you conduct research. Using the example of the health benefits of chocolate for middle-aged women (presented earlier in this chapter), let's say that you conduct the search and find that there are no studies on this topic in this population. You would then expand your search to see if the benefits of chocolate have been studied in other populations (such as males or young adults) and if there are sound explanations (theories) for how and why chocolate produces a beneficial effect.

For the purpose of demonstration, let's say that you have finished your search and have found several studies on the effect of chocolate on anxiety and on mood. It is important now to organize your articles in some meaningful way. For example, you could sort them according to the types of studies (e.g., systematic review, randomized controlled trial, or descriptive study); according to the population studied (e.g., children, adolescents, or young adults); or according to the outcome variables (e.g., anxiety and mood). You can usually obtain information from the abstract that will help you to sort. There are no hard and fast rules about sorting techniques. But as an example, consider that you have 10 studies: 3 in children, 4 in adolescents, and 3 in young adults. These age groups may be a good way to organize the studies. However, if all the studies are in children between the ages of 6 and 12, obviously you couldn't sort by this method and you would look for other ways to group the studies.

The next step is to evaluate, or appriase, the studies. Generally speaking, you review each study for its quality and strength of evidence (see Chapter 2 for levels of evidence), noting the strengths and weaknesses of each. You might be experienced in doing this or it might be a new skill for you. If it is new to you, you should seek guidance from an experienced researcher. Polit and Beck (2010) have produced a review protocol that you might find to be a useful guide for extracting the necessary information from each study. The benefit of using a protocol is that it you can systematically record information contained in a study in a concise manner. Some headings on a protocol that cue you to the information needed would include, for example, the full citation for the study, study design, sample, data collection techniques, method of data analysis, and your evaluation of the strength and weaknesses of the study. You can, of course, construct your own protocol, but you should be sure that it captures all of the necessary information from the study.

After you have evaluated all of the studies, another organizing strategy is to put the information from each study into a table. Experienced researchers find that they are able to put the information directly into a table and capture all the elements needed. As a neophyte researcher, you might not be able to do this as easily. A table enables you to see at a glance all the pertinent information and to compare the studies with one another. You can find examples of tables in Chapter 2 (see Figure 2.5) and Chapter 10 (see Figure 10.1). Or, if you choose to, you can design your own. What is important here, as with a protocol, is that all of the headings in the table cue you to insert the important information from your studies. When the information from all of the studies is inserted into the table, you can more easily see similarities and differences among the studies as well as any gaps in knowledge. This will help to prepare you to write the literature review section of your proposal.

For example, let's say you have constructed a table of studies on the topic of adult patient preferences for the color of nurses' uniforms. When you look at the "sample" section of the table, you notice that in all of the studies the racial breakdown of the sample consisted of mostly White men and woman. You may then conclude that what is unknown is the preference for uniform colors in a more racially diverse population (a gap in knowledge). If you work in a setting where the patient population is more racially diverse, conducting a study on their preference for uniform color would fill the gap in knowledge.

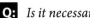 *Is it necessary to use a table to organize my studies?*

 Although it is not absolutely necessary, a table is very useful and can save a lot of time. It will also help you not to miss important information contained in the studies. The headings of the table should cue you as to what information should be plugged in. Although this may seem like more work at first, it will save you time when you write your literature review, and your review will be more organized.

Writing the Literature Review

The literature review lets the reader know what is known about your topic and builds the case for conducting your study. It is a good idea to start by identifying the strategy you used to conduct the search, including search terms (keywords) used, databases searched, the number of articles retrieved from each database, and the years searched. This lets the reader know how comprehensive the search was.

Next, you can establish headings based upon how you sorted your articles. For example, if you have organized your studies according to age groups, then your headings would be "Studies of Chocolate in Children," "Studies of Chocolate in Adolescents," and "Studies of Chocolate in Young Adults." If you have organized your studies according to types of studies, then your headings might be "Randomized Controlled Trials," "Correlational Studies," "Descriptive Studies," and so on.

Finally, for each section, write a short description of the studies and the findings. When you have written your descriptions, summarize all of the findings in one or two paragraphs. The literature review should end with a statement about the gap in knowledge, which could go something like this: "Although the benefits of chocolate in reducing anxiety and improving mood have been studied in other age groups, there are no studies on such benefits to middle-aged women. The proposed study is intended to fill this gap."

Try It Now!

Using the PICOT question format you learned in Chapter 2, identify two to four key concepts or search terms. Select an appropriate database and try a search. If you get too many "hits," try narrowing your search terms. Conversely, if you don't get any "hits," what do you think your next step will be? Hint: You might try alternative search terms, or you might have just identified an area ripe for research!

References

Coulter, P. (2012). What's the difference between a research article (or research study) and a review article? Retrieved from http://apus.libanswers.com/a.php?qid=153014

Polit, D. F. & Beck, C. T. (2010). *Essentials of nursing research: Appraising evidence for nursing practice* (7th ed.). Philadelphia: Wolters Kluwer Health Lippincott, Williams, & Wilkins.

Planning Your Study: Quantitative Research Designs

7

Christine Hedges

WHAT YOU'LL LEARN IN THIS CHAPTER

- Good research questions will determine the design you choose for your study.

- Two broad categories of quantitative design are experimental and non-experimental. Myriad research designs exist within each category.

- Assuring validity is important when designing a quantitative study.

- Staff nurses who are designing quantitative studies should consider various aspects of the their study and consult with an experienced researcher before deciding upon a design.

A finished product appears so seamless. When you attend a symphony, the sublime tones reach your senses in perfection, never hinting at the hours of orchestral rehearsal and preparation that came before. Likewise, your excellent nursing care appears effortless and expert to your patient—the patient does not see your educational preparation, nursing care plan, or practice guidelines that prepared you to provide expert care.

Think back to nursing school when you learned how to care for patients with chronic obstructive pulmonary disease (COPD). Your textbooks provided nursing care plans that included steps (nursing interventions), rationale (reason for the intervention), and expected outcomes (the result you expect). As a novice, you spent hours completing care plans prior to starting your clinical experience so that you had a plan for delivering expert care. You knew that you needed a plan in order to help your patient achieve normal breathing patterns, clear breath sounds, and effective gas exchange. And that individualized plan or blueprint drives the care you deliver to each patient every day.

There is design to all worthwhile endeavors; there is design to nursing; and there is design for the conduct of research. Research studies require a rigorous plan—a "blueprint," or design—to ensure that your study "works." This chapter explains quantitative research methods, including what types of questions are answered with quantitative methods, the various types of quantitative research designs, and what questions you should ask before choosing a design for your quantitative research.

Quantitative Versus Qualitative Research

Both quantitative and qualitative research methods involve design decisions. Qualitative research, which focuses on words to describe data, is covered in greater detail in Chapter 12. For example, a researcher who seeks to understand the experience of persons living with end stage heart failure would use a qualitative design (words). In this case the researcher would elicit descriptions and present the findings as narrative. By comparison, quantitative research methods use numerical data to describe or assess relationships between and among variables. For example, a researcher who wishes to examine the relationship between a client's stage of heart failure and their sleep quality would be use a quantitative design (numbers). In this case numbers are used to indicate the individual's stage of heart failure and to measure their sleep quality. Quantitative research methods are highly formal, objective, and systematic, and they rely upon objective statistical procedures for their analysis.

Your determination of whether to use quantitative, qualitative, or both (mixed methods) in your research study depends on many factors, including the purpose, aims, and research questions you want to answer. Choosing a research method should not be an arbitrary decision or personal preference any more than choosing a nursing care plan is without reason. The latter depends on your patient's individual diagnosis and problem list; the former depends on the research question you want to answer.

Q: *The nurse scientist in my hospital suggested that I do a qualitative study to answer my research question. I'm better with numbers, so I want to do a quantitative study. Does it really matter whether I choose quantitative or qualitative design for my study?*

A: Your choice of design depends on the question you asked, so your nurse scientist is assisting you to select the best design to answer your question. That said, another consideration is the knowledge and skills you need to conduct the study. If the study is best answered with a qualitative design and you don't have that experience, you should find someone with knowledge of qualitative methods to lead the study team. Or you might explore a different question related to your topic of interest that would lend itself to quantitative design.

Types of Research Questions Answered With Quantitative Methods

In my practice as a nurse scientist, I often consult with nurses and students who want to conduct research and need a little help getting started. They have passion for a topic and can discuss nearly everything that is known and unknown about the topic. "Great!" I say. "Now, what is *your* question?" This is often where the nurse or student gets stuck, which takes us back to the skills outlined in Chapter 3: asking a good clinical question. After you have accomplished that step, and you've performed your literature review and determined exactly what your research question is, or what hypothesis it is that you want to test, it is time to make decisions about how to answer the question.

In quantitative research, decisions focus on whether you want to:

- *Describe* phenomena of interest

- Assess for *differences* between or among groups or individuals

- Test *relationships* among variables

- Seek to explain *cause and effect interactions* between variables

- Test whether or not an *intervention* was effective or successful

Furthermore, there are a variety of research designs available, from simple to complex, depending on which method your research is following. The bottom line is that you want to choose the design that best answers your research question!

Quantitative Research Designs

This section examines some of the more common research designs you are likely to encounter as a clinical nurse researcher. There exist myriad design terms in quantitative research, but they are most easily understood when you consider the intent. For instance, do you intend to establish cause-and-effect in your study? Or do you intend to describe phenomena? One way of looking at design is to consider categories. The broadest categories are experimental and nonexperimental research designs.

Experimental Designs

Experimental designs seek to test the effectiveness of interventions and involve a high level of control and rigor. Experimental studies are concerned with cause and effect. Remember when you learned the terms *independent* and *dependent* variables? Recall that your independent variable (IV) was termed the "cause" and your dependent variable (DV) was the "effect." Establishing true cause and effect in human subject research can be challenging. One way to design a cause-and-effect study is to manipulate or control your independent variable in order to see if there is an effect on your dependent variable. For example, if you wanted to see if applying heat to the venipuncture site before inserting the intravenous cannulae resulted in less pain for the patient and a greater likelihood of accessing the vein first time, you could assign some subjects to receive the intervention of heat, while others receive usual care and do not get the application of heat. You are manipulating the independent variable of heat application.

When you consult a rating system for the hierarchy of evidence in evidence-based practice (EBP), have you noticed that true experiments—or randomized controlled trials (RCT)—are always at the top of the hierarchy? (See Table 2.3 in Chapter 2.) This is because a true experiment involves a great deal of *control*, *manipulation* of the intervention (how is this new intervention delivered), and *randomization*—like flipping a coin (some subjects are randomized to the experimental group, whereas others are randomized to the control group). The two groups are then compared. Because of this high level of control, RCTs are the strongest design to support cause-and-effect relationships (Melnyk & Fineout-Overholt, 2011). RCTs are commonly seen in clinical trials research involving large sample sizes and multisite studies. For this reason, they were not seen commonly in nursing research, although that is changing.

> **Example of an experimental study design:** The COPE intervention for caregivers of patients with heart failure (McMillan, Small, Haley, Zambroski, & Buck, 2013)
>
> Description of this experimental design: Two-group comparative experimental design. The control group consisted of patient-caregiver dyads who received usual care; the treatment group consisted of dyads who received usual care plus an intervention that supported family caregivers and consisted of creativity, optimism, planning, and expert information—known as the COPE educational intervention.

As an alternative to an experimental design, researchers will conduct what looks very much like an experimental design but is lacking one of the elements. Generally, there is either no comparison group or no randomization. This type of design is known as a *quasiexperimental design*.

> **Example of a quasiexperimental design:** The effect of hand massage on preoperative anxiety in ambulatory surgery patients (Brand, Munroe, & Gavin, 2013)
>
> Description of this quasiexperimental design: Quasiexperimental design with pretest and posttest evaluations. Subjects were non-randomly assigned to either the hand massage intervention or the control group (usual care).

One reason there needs to be control in an experimental study is because of those pesky little variables known as *extraneous* or *intervening* variables. These are variables that are not the IV, but exert an effect on the DV! And the best way to manage these is to control them (or hold them constant) through your design. For example, if you want to design a study to determine if playing 20 minutes of relaxing music reduces your critical care patient's anxiety level, what extraneous variables would you need to consider? Perhaps your patient doesn't like your choice of music. Suppose the patient is in pain. Perhaps the patient is watching a distressing news report on the TV while the music is being delivered. Each of these could exert an effect on your DV of anxiety without you being aware!

Now think of how you might control the influence of the extraneous variables: Your protocol could give the patient a choice of types of music; you could exclude patients who are in pain; and you could specify that TV must be off during the delivery of the music therapy! Furthermore, you make these adjustments because you know that the extraneous variables, if not considered carefully in your design, could affect the *validity* of your study.

Researchers often call these *threats* to the validity of research designs because they are factors that could account for rival or alternative explanations of your results. Sometimes these rival explanations are referred to as *limitations* of the study and are addressed at the conclusion of the research when reporting the results (Nieswiadomy, 2012). Researchers who undertake studies that examine the effects of independent variables on dependent variables are cognizant of what are known as threats to the internal and external validity of the study, as any one of these could alter the precision, dependability, or truthfulness of the results (Lobiondo-Wood & Haber, 2006).

Q: *I am designing a study to see if delivery of our new preoperative hip surgery educational booklet when compared to our usual 10-minute hip surgery video results in less anxiety for patients about to undergo elective hip surgery. Are there any other variables that I need to consider in the design of my study?*

A: Yes! You will need to consider the reading level of the new booklet and the educational level of the patients who will be reading it. You may also want to consider primary language spoken by your subjects and cultural competency of the new reading materials as each of these could affect your dependent variable. Can you think of any others?

Internal validity. The internal validity of a study becomes threatened when something other than the independent variable accounts for the effect on the dependent variable. For instance, returning to the example of studying the effect of 20 minutes of relaxing music on the anxiety of critical care patients, suppose that rather than randomly selecting patients for the study, you only select patients who previously enjoyed listening to relaxing music. This sample selection would be biased toward supporting your hypothesis. This threat to internal validity is called *selection bias* because now the selection of certain types of patients may have influenced your dependent variable.

External validity. The external validity of a study becomes threatened when the findings of the study cannot be extended, transferred, or generalized beyond this research to another sample or setting. For instance, an interesting threat to the external validity of an experimental study is something known as the *Hawthorne effect* or *reactive effect*, in which a subject may behave differently if the subject knows that he/she is being observed or studied. For example, if you knew that you were being observed for handwashing as a subject in a study on hand hygiene, do you think your behavior might be affected? Could the results obtained in that study then be extended or generalized to handwashing behaviors in another setting?

Threats to validity. There are several different types of threats to both the internal and external validity of studies. See Table 7.1 for a full list of threats to study validity.

Clearly it is difficult to accomplish complete control of extraneous variables in most nursing research as it is not conducted in a laboratory setting but in the human setting—the clinical environment. This is why many nursing studies fall into the category of non-experimental research.

Table 7.1   Threats to Study Validity

Internal Validity	Threats to Internal Validity	Description
At issue: Is it the independent variable (or something else) that causes an effect on or influences the dependent variable?	History	An event occurred during the study which may affect results
	Maturation	Subjects change (grow or mature) during course of study
	Testing	Repeated administration of same test or tool influences or "primes" subjects' responses
	Instrumentation	Measurement tools may be subject to inaccuracies (e.g. calibration, administration)
	Mortality	Subjects are lost to follow-up
	Selection Bias	Subjects were not selected or enrolled objectively or randomly.
External Validity	**Threats to External Validity**	**Description**
At issue: Can the findings from this study be generalized to another population?	Hawthorne Effect (reactive effect of the test)	Subjects' behavior changes due to knowledge of being studied
	Measurement effects	Pretesting affects the post-test, thereby altering the generalizability of results
	Selection effects	Subjects selected are not representative; threatens the generalizability of results

Nonexperimental Designs

Nonexperimental designs are used more commonly in nursing research that involves human subjects and phenomena that are not really amenable to manipulation, either for practical or ethical reasons. For example, if you were interested in the phenomenon of workplace aggression in the emergency department, you could hardly design an experimental study and plan to deliver an "intervention" of aggression!

In quantitative studies with nonexperimental designs, the researcher will seek to learn more about a phenomenon (such as workplace aggression) by describing it, or comparing it with another sample or setting, or looking for associations between the phenomenon and other variables. Nonexperimental designs exist primarily to *describe, test relationships*, or *compare*; but never to determine cause-and-effect or to test the effectiveness of interventions. Some common types of studies seen in nonexperimental designs are the following:

- Survey studies

- Correlational studies

- Comparative studies

Survey studies. Surveys are one type of descriptive study often used to seek opinions, attitudes, health care needs, knowledge deficits, and barriers and facilitators to practice, among other things. Survey research has traditionally occurred by paper-and-pencil format, but is appearing more in an electronic medium (see Chapter 17). Survey research is descriptive, and, as such, the analysis is limited to descriptive techniques. But results obtained from studies designed with descriptive survey research can provide information that leads to development of more complex study designs in the future.

> **Example of survey research study:** A statewide survey identifying perceived barriers to hospice use in nursing homes (Tarzian & Hoffman, 2006)

> Description of the survey methods: Respondents included employees from licensed hospices who participated in a telephone survey and employee respondents from licensed nursing homes who participated in a mailed survey.

Correlational studies. Suppose you want to compare or elicit an association or relationship between and among phenomena. In experimental studies, you seek to determine whether the IV exerts an effect on the DV. In correlational studies, the nurse researcher suspects that there might be a relationship or an association between variables, rather than cause-and-effect.

For example, you might wonder if the functional decline you observe during hospitalization of many elderly patients is related to the amount of time they spend in bed. Rather than designing an experimental study to test the hypothesis, and randomizing patients to an intervention, you choose to describe the phenomenon as it exists. In this study, you would collect data on the variable of "time in bed" and also collect data on "functional decline" (perhaps your unit is collecting data on a functional status or activities of daily living scale). You might then see if a correlation or association exists to answer your research question (*Is time in bed related to functional decline in hospitalized elders?*) or to support a hypothesis (*Greater amount of time in bed is related to greater functional decline in hospitalized elders*).

> **Example of correlational study:** Relationships of assertiveness, depression, and social support among older nursing home residents (Segal, 2005)
>
> Description of correlational study: Participants completed self-report measures of assertiveness, depression, and social support. Results were analyzed for relationships between/among the three study variables.

Comparative studies. There are times when using a nonexperimental research design when you may want to compare groups of patients to see if differences exist between groups in a research study. In this case, you might want to conduct a comparative study.

Again using the example of examining functional decline in the elderly, suppose that your hospital has an Acute Care of the Elderly (ACE) unit and some elderly patients are admitted to the ACE unit whereas others are admitted to a general medical-surgical unit. You want to compare subjects on the two units on the variable of functional decline, and so you decide to design a comparative study. Comparative studies might sound a lot like experimental designs (after all, you are making comparisons in experiments). The difference between the nonexperimental, comparative study and the experimental design is in the manipulation of the IV (Nieswiadomy, 2012). In the comparative study, there is no manipulation of the IV, as in this example you are looking at characteristics of the two intact units. In an experimental design, the researcher would manipulate the IV.

> **Example of comparative research study:** Graduated compression stockings in hospitalized postoperative patients: Correctness of usage and size (Winslow & Brosz, 2008)
>
> Description of this comparative study: The researchers used a descriptive, comparative design to compare leg measurements against manufacturer sizing to see if stockings were being used/applied correctly.

Descriptive survey, correlational, and descriptive comparative research occupies a lower level on the evidence hierarchy as no causal relationships can be inferred. However, these types of nonexperimental designs might be the most appropriate to answer the research question and should still apply the same rigorous criteria expected in any research study.

Q: *Sometimes I have trouble identifying the independent and dependent variables, especially in correlational studies. Help!*

A: You are not alone. Identifying the IV and DV is easiest in experimental studies where there is delivery of an intervention and examination of an outcome. This is not always the case in studies about relationships between and among variables. It is not always clear "which came first." For example, when examining the relationship between stress and anxiety, the temporal relationship is unclear. However, the relationship between smoking and lung cancer is clear; you would not consider that lung cancer resulted in smoking!

Other Elements to Consider in Design

The number of groups in your study is an important design consideration, too. Often the researcher needs to consider whether they will be making comparisons with only *one group* of subjects at two different times—for example, patients before and after their hip surgeries. At other times, your study might involve comparing *two or more different groups* of subjects—for example, male patients and female patients, or mothers who breastfeed and mothers who bottle feed their infants.

There may also be a time element of your proposed research design. There are times when your question requires you to "look back" and see what has happened in the past, and there are times when your research question can be answered only by "looking forward" to see what will happen in the future. Chart review studies are a good way of looking back and answering a question through a *retrospective* method. Sometimes this method is called *ex post facto*. At other times, you may want to follow a subject looking forward or through a *prospective* method, to see if a certain condition develops given a set of circumstances. Very often, prospective research involves examining a subject at several points over time in a *longitudinal design*, as opposed to examining at only one point in time in a *cross-sectional design*. See Table 7.2 for an overview of common quantitative research designs.

Table 7.2   Overview of Quantitative Research Designs

Broad Category	Examples of Designs	Features
Experimental designs	True experiment (RCT)	Controlled trial with randomization.
	Quasiexperimental	Controlled trial without randomization.
Nonexperimental designs	Survey research studies	Surveys elicit people's opinions, attitudes, and beliefs, among other things.
	Correlational studies	Examines associations or relationships between variables. May be descriptive or predictive.
	Comparative studies	Compares differences between intact groups. No manipulation of IV.
	Case study	Single subject or single group examined in depth.
	Methodological studies	Used to test new instruments for validity and reliability.

Choosing a Quantitative Method

This chapter has covered some of the basics of quantitative design. As you read more research studies, you will become familiar with more designs. We advise you to consult one of the research texts in the reference list at the end of this chapter for a more detailed description of any design with which you are not familiar. This will not only help you to choose a design for your planned research, but also it will help you to discern levels of evidence when evaluating research to put into practice!

If you are planning a study, you should plan a consultation with a nurse scientist, statistician, or someone else with experience who can assist you to identify the most appropriate research design to answer your research question. Before scheduling an appointment with the expert, there are several questions you and your team should ask yourselves in preparation for your meeting:

1. What is the purpose of my/our research? (Is it to describe, compare, or to determine cause and effect?)

2. Will there be an intervention? Will the investigator have control over the intervention? (If so, perhaps you will need help with an experimental or quasiexperimental design.)

3. If a comparison is to be made, who will be the subjects/participants in the study? Will you be comparing a single group of subjects before and after? Or will you be comparing two or more different group of subjects?

4. Will you answer your question by looking back in time (are you considering chart review, for instance) or looking forward in time (following a group of subjects with a particular condition and seeing what develops)?

5. Will you be studying or surveying your subjects only once or on multiple occasions?

These are all important questions to ask as you formulate your design. Taking the time to do it well will pay off; a clear design plan will lead quite elegantly into your proposed data analysis, just as a clear nursing care plan informs the precise care you will deliver!

Writing the Design Section of Your Proposal

The design section is actually one of the easiest sections of your proposal to write—assuming you have done your work! Under the Methods section, you will state the design you intend to use. The design should flow logically from your review of the literature, your purpose, aims, and your research questions or hypotheses. Sometimes you will see it listed simply as "Design," and other times it may be stated as "Design, Sample, and Setting." In either case, the person reading your proposal should clearly see exactly what you intend to do; the Design section is the "blueprint" for the study. Your purpose and aims, research questions, and hypotheses will even have "clues" as to what type of design you will use. For example:

The study will examine the *difference*...	Comparative design
Is there an *association* between X and Y?	Correlational design
Does the implementation of X *cause* Y?	Experimental design
The purpose of this survey is to *describe*...	Descriptive design

Your proposal for your study design should clearly state what you are going to do in very specific language. For example, if you are doing a comparison, are you using a pretest and posttest design with one group of subjects, or are you comparing two different groups and examining them one time? Describe any factors that may present limitations or threaten the validity of your study and describe how you will control them. For example, if there is an intervention, describe how your control group will be treated in comparison to your study group. Will they receive the same care in all regards except for the intervention? Be sure to describe the time elements of your design and let the reader know if you intend to study your subjects looking forward or study them by gathering data that has already been collected or is available to you, such as through medical records or nursing documentation sources. If you are very clear about your design, your reader is then prepared for the next section on how you will select your sample and how you intend to measure your variables, as it will follow logically.

Try It Now!

Your research team would like to study the effect of open visitation on family and nurse satisfaction in your ICU. Your ICU committee has agreed that a trial period of open visitation could be accommodated for your study. Write your research question (refer to Chapter 4 for help); then fill out the worksheet below for determining your design.

Design exercise: Before meeting with your research mentor, nurse scientist, or statistician, you and your team should try completing as much of this worksheet as possible.

Fill in the blanks:

The purpose statement or aim of our study is _____.

Our research question is _____.

   Or

Our hypothesis is _____.

Now underline key "clue" words (describe, compare, etc.).

Will there be an intervention? (Are you doing something to your subjects?) Yes or No

Who will be our subjects? _____

Is there more than one group of subjects? Yes or No

Will you be making any comparisons between or among groups of subjects? Yes or No

How many times will you be studying them? _____

Will you be looking at data from the past or following subjects forward? _____

Our research design is _____.

Figure 7.1   Design exercise

References

Brand, L. R,, Munroe, D. J., & Gavin, J. (2013). The effect of hand massage on preoperative anxiety in ambulatory surgery patients. *AORN Journal, 97*(6), 708–717.

Lobiondo-Wood, G., & Haber, J. (2006). *Nursing research: Methods and critical appraisal for evidence-based practice* (6th ed.). St. Louis: Mosby Elsevier.

McMillan, S., Small, B., Haley, W., Zambroski, C., & Buck, H. (2013). The COPE intervention for caregivers of patients with heart failure. *Journal of Hospice and Palliative Nursing, 15*(4), 196–206.

Melnyk, B., & Fineout-Overholt, E. (2011). *Evidence-based practice in nursing & healthcare* (2nd ed.). Philadephia: Wolters Kluwer Health, Lippincott, Williams, & Wilkins.

Nieswiedomy, R. (2012). *Foundations of nursing research* (6th ed.). Boston: Pearson Health Science.

Segal, D. (2005). Relationships of assertiveness, depression, and social support among older nursing home residents. *Behavior Modification, 29*(4), 689–685.

Tarzian, A,. & Hoffman, D. (2006). A statewide survey identifying perceived barriers to hospice use in nursing homes. *Journal of Hospice and Palliative Care Nursing, 8*(6), 328–337.

Winslow, E. H., & Brosz, D. L. (2008). Graduated compression stockings in hospitalized post-operative patients: Correctness of usage and size. *American Journal of Nursing, 108*(9), 40–50.

> *"Somewhere, something incredible*
> *is waiting to be known."*
>
> –Dr. Carl Sagan

Methods: Choosing Your Sample for Quantitative Studies

8

Pamela Willson
Karen Stonecypher

- You'll need to choose a sample for your study by identifying characteristics that represent your study population.

- Then, you can design a sampling plan for your study that meets the specific criteria for either a probability or nonprobability sample.

- To calculate the number of participants (sample size), you will need to use the significance level, power, and effect size found from previous research studies.

Clinical research begins with a research question concerning a characteristic, a health condition, learning need, or outcome for a particular patient population. As nurses, we often want to know which teaching method, intervention, or type of product leads to the best outcomes or results for our patients. We may want to know which health promotion nursing intervention has the highest patient adherence for regular exercise or which antiseptic preparation kit supports lower blood culture infection rates. We are looking for evidence to change nursing practice.

For example, the emergency department (ED) has an 8% blood culture contamination rate. Thirty percent of all hospital blood cultures are drawn in the ED. All ED patients with a fever were selected as the intervention group to change the evidence-based practice (EBP) of cleaning the skin prior to drawing blood cultures. The ED patients represent a *sample* of about a third of the entire hospital patient *population* who had blood cultures drawn. The sample is a subset or portion of the larger population group that contains all possible cases (people, objects, events). The ED blood culture contamination rates can be compared to the remaining hospital contamination rates to determine if the new evidence-based skin preparation procedure was an effective intervention. This chapter reviews specific methods for choosing your sample and describes how an adequately sized representative sample is determined.

Choosing a Representative Sample: Inclusion and Exclusion Criteria

Before you can begin recruiting or selecting the sample participants, you need to ask yourself, "What are the characteristics of the population under study?" After you identify those distinctive characteristics—such as gender, age, ethnicity, race, health status, education, or any other aspect that makes up the population—you can choose a representative sample. The characteristics can be determined by answering the questions of who, what, and where for your research question. List the population characteristics and then ask:

- "How can I make sure that my sample is representative or has the same features as the population?"

- "What population characteristics would mask, confound, or interfere with the study outcomes?"

For example, if you want to learn what nurses might do to prevent methicillin-resistant staphylococcus aureus (MRSA) spread in the surgical intensive care unit (SICU), one (1) of the *inclusion criteria* for the sample would be to choose only patients admitted to the SICU. Other inclusion criteria would be patients who (2) had surgery, (3) were adults, and (4) were patients who remained in SICU for at least 24 hours.

Situational and patient characteristics that might produce erroneous or biased study results if included in the study are nonsurgical overflow patients, patients having MRSA prior to surgery, children, or patients not remaining in the unit long enough to experience the nursing intervention of a daily bath with antibacterial soap. Therefore, to control for unwanted influences you would not include them in this study. The *exclusion criteria* for the study would be (1) patients who are nonsurgical, (2) patients who are MRSA positive on admission, (3) patients who are under age 18, and (4) patients with an SICU stay less than 24 hours. If age might affect the study results, then by excluding young patients from participating you would be able to control for the age variation influence (differences between old and young patients that are caused by age).

Enrolling a representative sample ensures that the study results can be applied or generalized to the larger target population.

Sampling Methods in Quantitative Studies

After you have determined who you will include, what characteristics the subjects should possess to be similar to the population, and where the study will take place, you are ready to start devising the sampling plan. The *sampling plan* describes:

- The method used to choose the sample

- What measurements will be taken

- How many subjects/participants (units, cases) you will need in the sample

- Who is responsible for obtaining the data

Review the following probability and nonprobability sampling methods with examples of each strategy so that you may choose between sampling schemes to match the purpose of your study.

Probability Sampling

Probability sampling is the method of choosing an equivalent representation (a random sample) of the whole population. In other words, the sample characteristics are the same as the population's because each person in the population has an opportunity of being selected for the sample. The various types of probability sampling include:

- Simple random sample

- Stratified random sampling

- Proportionate stratified sampling

- Systematic sampling

- Cluster sampling

The following sections describe these sampling types in more detail.

Simple random sample. A simple random sample is a common approach used to select the sample where every individual has an equal chance of being selected. Selecting your sample randomly means you were not biased (prejudiced) in your sample selection. In other words you did not pick your friends or your healthy patients to be in your study so that your results would be good. The randomness of the selection process minimizes the effect of errors made by the selection. The randomly selected sample is more representative of the entire population.

To create a simple random sample, start by numbering the list of all possible subjects in the population (e.g., a list of all nurses belonging to a nursing organization or the number of accredited hospitals with more than 200 beds in the United States). Then refer to a random number table to identify a list of numbers. In turn, you will match the generated list of numbers with the enumerated population list (sampling frame) to pick the subjects/units for the sample.

 Where can I find a random number table?

 You can find random number tables in almost any statistics textbook, or you can use a web-based random number table such as the one at Random.org (http://www.random.org).

For example, let's say you need five more RNs to cover for a holiday, but you want to fill the openings fairly. If you want to draw a simple random sample from RNs who are available to work, you could make a numbered list of all RNS (e.g., 1–Maggie Jones, 2–Tom Smith, etc.). Next, run the random number generator. Let's suppose the following numbers came up: 3, 12, 1, 8, 2. You would then select nurse 3, nurse 12, and so on until you have collected the five randomly selected RNs needed for the holiday coverage.

Stratified random sampling. It is beneficial to use a stratified random sampling technique any time your population has characteristics that may affect the outcomes you are studying (e.g., education level). Similar to the simple random sample, you break down a *stratified random sampling* into categories, or groups, with each group numbered. Then you draw a random sample from each group. For example, you might first divide the population by gender (men and women), or registered nurses by education (associate, baccalaureate, and diploma degrees), or patients by disease severity (stage I, II, III carcinoma). Then each group is numbered before using a random number generator to choose a portion of the sample from each group. If you want to compare senior nursing students' educational program type with their passage of the licensure exam, you could obtain one-third of the sample from each of the three program types (associate, baccalaureate, and diploma degrees) to come up with the total sample.

Proportionate stratified sampling. A proportionate stratified sample maintains the same proportion or percentage of subjects within each category, assuring that each grouping is equally represented in your study. You may choose to use a *proportionate stratified sampling* by selecting subjects in the same percentages by program types who are taking the licensure exam in the United States in a given year (e.g., 56% associate, 42% baccalaureate, and 2% diploma degree program students). It is necessary to know the stratum, or group-defining variable, before the study begins and to balance the proportions to an acceptable norm (i.e., National Council of State Boards of Nursing report of pass rates).

Systematic sampling. When you use *systematic sampling*, every k^{th} eligible participant (i.e., k = 3rd or k = 10th case listed) is drawn from the enumerated list. To improve the representativeness of the sample, you can calculate a sampling interval by dividing the population size (N) by the sample size (n). For example, the sampling interval of every 10th subject of the sampling frame of a 1,000-person population would be chosen to end up with a sample of 100 subjects (k = N/n). Remember you determine your starting point for the subject selection by randomly selecting the first participant and from that point forward select every k^{th} subject (Yount, 2006). This is a very useful method for large sampling frames, such as chart reviews of a particular type of patient (e.g., diabetics) seen in your hospital during the past 5 years.

Q: *I've seen both capital* N *and lowercase* n *in articles that I read. What is* N?

A: N refers to the size of the sample. Just remember that *N* equals the Number of people in your study who responded to your questionnaire or agree to be in your study. You would not include the number of people you asked but who declined to be in your study in your sample size calculation. You would, however, track and report the nonresponders. The lowercase *n* represents the number of participants in the subgroups of your sample, for example, N = 20 (sample size) made up of n = 10 women and n = 10 men.

Cluster sampling. Cluster sampling is used when the population is very large and a random sample is desired. Random sampling methods require that each member of the population is known or listed for the researcher. When that is impossible or requires too much time or money, you might need to employ *cluster sampling*. The Federal Health Care System is a suitable population for successive random cluster sampling of the various medical centers across the United States. First, all facilities would be listed, and a random sample of the facilities (cluster) would be made. Cluster sampling is a multistep process and is sometimes called *multistage sampling* because you randomly select groups (e.g., hospitals or colleges) and not individuals. After you have selected the group, you make the decision of how to choose the sample from within each group. Do you use all the members or a portion of the members? If you use a portion of the group members, you can maintain your random selection by double randomizing your sample. A double randomized sample is obtained after you choose the cluster sample, by drawing another random sample (simple, stratified, or systematic) for each of the cluster facilities.

We have just described probability sampling—simple, stratified, systematic, and cluster sampling. Randomization is key to building representative samples (Yount, 2006). Probability samples enable the investigator to use inferential statistics to determine the sampling error and to calculate the estimated sample size. If randomly sampling the population is not possible, a nonprobability method is employed.

Nonprobability Sampling

You may find it necessary to use a *nonprobability sampling* method when it is impossible or difficult to obtain lists of the population. For example, it might be difficult to obtain a list of all American nurses who completed online education in the past 12 months. The inability to provide the entire population an equal chance of selection into the sample decreases the likelihood of a credible or representative sample. However, strategies that improve the investigator's objectivity into participant selection reduce the inherent investigator and systematic bias of nonprobability sampling.

One technique used to decrease bias when random sampling is not possible is to use a nonprobability sample and then randomly assign the participants to the various groups. Let's return to the example presented earlier of the study investigating blood culture contamination in the ED. All the patients who come to the ED with fever would represent a nonprobability sample because they were not randomly selected. However, you could randomly assign the patients to one of the two interventions (i.e., betadine or chlorhexidine). Random assignment ensures that each participant has an equal chance to be chosen for either intervention.

Q: *Is there a difference between random sampling and random assignment?*

A: Yes! Random sampling is probability sampling using a method such as a random number generator to assure that each individual has an equal chance of being selected. Random assignment occurs in nonprobability sampling; the sample was not selected randomly, but the researcher used a method like flipping a coin to assign subjects to one group or another.

There are three types of nonprobability sampling:

- Convenience sampling

- Snowball sampling

- Quota sampling

The types of nonprobability sampling will be reviewed in detail to guide your sampling strategies.

Convenience sampling. *Convenience sampling* is making use of available subjects; for that reason it is sometimes referred to as an *accidental sample*. Nursing studies use convenience sampling because of the availability to patient groups at clinics, hospitals, and other health care-related sites. One way to minimize investigator bias is to institute a consecutive sampling plan, whereby every patient coming to the site who meets the study criteria is recruited, rather than the investigator consciously or unconsciously judging which patient to approach for the study. When convenience sampling is used, the study results might only reflect the participants studied, and the results might not be generalizable to the target population.

Q: *Can a study that used convenience sampling provide evidence for practice change?*

A: Yes, a well-organized and ample study that used a convenience sample can provide evidence for practice change within the organization where the sample was drawn. However, you should take caution when generalizing the findings for practice change to the larger population, as the sample population might not be homogenous. Review the research article to make sure the investigators took measures to counter the nonrandomness of the sample selection, such as having a consecutive sample.

Snowball sampling. *Snowball sampling* recruits participants by asking knowledgeable subjects to identify other members of the target population so they can be recruited into your sample. Snowballing, or *chain/referral sampling*, is helpful for finding subjects when no list is available, such as persons who were victims of hurricane Katrina, homeless persons, or elders without caregivers. Snowballing begins when the investigator identifies a few subjects, and then the initial subjects identify other persons who also meet the study criteria for recruitment. For example, a widower was recruited for a study about care partners, and after his interview he was asked if he knew of other community members who lived alone who might be interested in participating in the study. The investigator contacts the suggested persons and determines their interest and eligibility for the study.

Quota sampling. Like convenience sampling, *quota sampling* begins with available subjects but specifically recruits subjects to address representativeness of the population. Quota sampling could be used if you are looking at the cultural preference in nutritional counseling at a prenatal clinic where the patients are 50% Asian, 10% Hispanic, 20% African American, and 20% Caucasian. The investigator wants to balance the ethnic proportion of the sample to match that of the population. He or she would divide the sample size of 100 to include 50 Asian, 10 Hispanic, 20 African-American, and 20 Caucasian subjects to make sure there are ample subjects in each independent variable category (ethnicity) to allow for statistical analysis.

Convenience, snowball, and quota sampling methods draw samples that often do not represent the population. It is likely that some segment of the population will be systematically under represented because the participants were not available to recruit into your convenience sample. Unfortunately, under or over representation of a sample variable may bias the study results and conclusions. The researcher should identify and control for extraneous (confounding) variables to improve representativeness of the sample (e.g., make the extraneous variable an exclusion criteria). If the population has variation in their characteristics (heterogeneous), you should take steps to make sure the sample is similar (heterogeneous). In the study example about cultural preferences for prenatal care, two different community clinics could be selected to capture a more culturally rich sample and lower the potential selection bias.

Estimating Your Sample Size

One of the questions that every clinical nurse researcher asks concerning samples is "How many subjects do I need for my study?" Sample size estimation is a topic that can leave many a neophyte researcher running for the door, so let us calm your fears by saying a sample size calculation is an educated guess. That said, how do you decide how many subjects are *enough*? How many subjects will be needed so that you can safely defend the results of your study?

There are both practical considerations and scientific considerations in this estimated guess. The practical considerations might center around how many subjects you have access to and resources to study (after all, you probably don't have funds to study thousands of subjects). The scientific consideration is the more important one: How certain do you want to be of the results? Let's look at the latter. The scientific approach to the estimation of sample size is to use mathematical formulas to determine the number of subjects needed to detect a statistically significant finding, if there is one (Hedges & Bliss-Holtz, 2006; see Chapter 11 for more on statistical significance.)

Determining a sample size depends on three things:

- Significance level (alpha level)

- Power

- Effect size

Let's break down each of these factors.

Significance level. *Significance level* is something you are probably already familiar with. It is the likelihood—usually set in a percentage—that something other than "chance" caused your results. In most nursing studies the alpha, or *p* value, is set at .05, meaning that there is only a 5% chance that the results obtained were found by chance. Put another way, if the *p* value falls below .05, you are 95% confident that that you have not falsely accepted results as "true" when in fact they were "false." This is known as a Type I error.

Error Types

Here are the two error types explained in simple terms:

- **Type I error:** With a Type I error, you think your treatment (or intervention) *did* work when in fact it *didn't* (potential for instituting an unwarranted change).

- **Type II error:** With a Type II error, you think your treatment (or intervention) *didn't* work when, in fact, it *did* (a potential missed opportunity).

Which error—Type I or Type II—is more serious, depends on the clinical circumstances.

Power. The next parameter to discuss is *power*, which is probably a new term to you. Power is your confidence in saying that the research findings are really correct—it is your certainty that the effect of the study, if it exists, will be found (Hedges & Bliss-Holtz, 2006). Power is expressed as a decimal, and .80 (80% certainty) is often used in nursing studies. Are you beginning to see why this is a "guess"? With statistical significance set at .05 and power at .80, only the effect size remains to be determined in order to calculate the sample size.

Effect size. The final number needed is something called *effect*. Effect is the magnitude, or size, of the effect of an intervention (Hedges & Bliss-Holtz, 2006). The effect size (ES) tells you how strong the relationship is between the population's dependent and independent variables; the most common ES in nursing studies has a range of .20 to .40 (Polit & Beck, 2008). These three numbers, when entered into a formula (known as a *power analysis*), can produce a mathematical estimation of a fourth number, the sample size—the number of participants needed for your study. (See Table 8.1.)

Table 8.1   Relationship Between Significance Level, Effect Size, Power, and Sample Size

Component	Impact on Sample Size
The significance level desired (also known as the alpha level)	Although the maximum significance level usually accepted is α = .05, in some studies this may be set lower—for example, to α = .01. The implication of this is that the lower the "acceptable" significance level, the larger the sample size will need to be.
The effect size of the intervention being investigated	As mentioned, the smaller the effect of an intervention is, the harder it will be to detect. The implication of this is that the smaller the effect size, the larger the sample will need to be.
The power level desired	By convention, the power of a study expresses the chance of obtaining a significant finding if it exists. The higher the power of a study, the larger the sample will need to be.

Reprinted with permission from Hedges, C., & Bliss-Holtz, J. (2006). Not too big, not too small, but just right: The dilemma of sample size estimation. AACN Advanced Critical Care, 17(3), 341-344.

Where the numbers come from. You might be thinking, "Where do I get these numbers?" Good question! This is another instance where you are strongly advised to talk with your statistician or nurse scientist before beginning your study. Come to your meeting with the statistician with some thoughtful information about what kind of results you hope to find. For instance, if previous studies or your own pilot data have been conducted on your topic, bring them with you. This will give the statistician some idea of how large an effect you hope to find. And think about how much risk you are willing to take to accept some error. Do the "conventions" of alpha .05 and power of .80 suffice for your study? Or do you want to accept less error?

> ### Resources for Calculating Sample Size
>
> As you have been taught throughout this book, use your resources (biostatisticians, nurse scientists, experienced research mentors). There are also online resources for calculating sample size such as:
>
> - G*Power: http://www.psycho.uni-duesseldorf.de/abteilungen/aap/gpower3/
> - Interactive Statistical Calculating Pages: http://statpages.org/
> - Statistical Solutions: http://statpages.org/

Sampling Suggestions

The previous section provides a background on the three parameters (significance level, power, and effect size) necessary for sample size calculations. However, your proposed study calculations might call for more subjects than the resources you have—either too much time or money, or too few accessible subjects. Underpowered studies with too few subjects are at risk of a Type II error (false negative results when indeed your nursing intervention did have a significant finding) because the number of participants was too small to mathematically determine a statistically significant difference. If you find yourself in a similar situation, you should consider the following sampling recommendations (DeMuth, 2008):

- Understand as much as you can about the target population (i.e., what are their characteristics?)
- Know about your sampling frame (i.e., does my list represent the population?)
- Use a sampling method that captures the population's study characteristics (i.e., would a stratified random sample be more effective?)

Other general rules to abide by are to use as large a sample as possible for survey and correlational research designs. Samples of 1,000 to 1,200 subjects from populations greater than 100,000 usually do not increase the statistical accuracy of the study, and samples smaller than 200 to 300 subjects often lead to wide confidence intervals that do not lend to subsample analyses (Hoskins & Mariano, 2004). The time spent up front preparing for your study's sample size is time well spent. A statistician or experienced nurse researcher can assist you if the effect size cannot be specified or if the reported sample variances cannot be determined.

Using Chart Review Studies and Preexisting Data

Using chart review studies and working with preexisting datasets can be challenging as the data was often collected for clinical reasons and not research—or, more specifically, it was not collected for your research question. For retrospective studies, after developing the research question, you must take care to clearly define the study variables before proceeding to scan the records to determine the feasibility of conducting your study (Gearing, Mian, Barber, & Ickowicz, 2006).

With a glossary of variable definitions and a familiarity with the medical chart, you need to devise a uniform data abstraction tool. An *abstraction tool* lists all the study variables and the variables are listed in the order they are found in the medical record/dataset. (The abstraction tool may be either a pen-and-paper form or an electronic tool; there are several available data abstraction software programs.) Use of the abstraction tool enhances completeness and reduces errors during data entry.

Q: *I want to study patients' functional status, but no data on the chart is labeled "functional status." What could we do?*

A: The nurses might document activities of daily living (ADLs) daily for each patient, using a standardized template in the electronic medical record. ADLs can be social (support, home therapy), psychological (cognitive assessment, mental status), and physical (nutrition, balance, vision, hearing). Some examples of ADLs for a study regarding physical functioning might be the patient's ability to feed him- or herself or ambulation and balance.

You need to develop guidelines and procedures for abstraction, for guiding and training the abstractors so as to improve inter-rater reliability (Gearing et al., 2006). For example, you may be interested in the quality of life of your patient population prior to the implementation of the new telemedicine service. If you look retrospectively at a dataset your clinic has maintained and there is a data point for health status from a standardized quality of life instrument, you must decide if "health status" answers your research question.

You must develop a sampling plan, identify a sampling frame, and calculate a sampling size. Sampling methods often used for retrospective studies are convenience, quota, and systematic sampling. Patient variables are collected for subjects meeting the inclusion and exclusion criteria for a specific timeframe, or a predetermined number of cases by diagnosis or every k^{th} case is selected from the dataset. A pilot study should precede the full study to allow for adjustments in the data collection guideline and procedures, inclusion and exclusion criteria, and to determine the amount and solutions for missing data.

Retrospective studies are perfect first steps in preparing for a larger study. The pilot outcomes can help the researcher evaluate the data collection tool, sampling technique, and abstractor training, as well as provide the data for the larger studies' sample size power analysis. Additionally, retrospective chart review/dataset studies can reveal a wealth of clinical information that can inform nursing practice.

Q: *I've decided to do a pilot study before starting a large study. How many participants do I need in my pilot study?*

A: In general, you will need to go through the same sample size estimation for your pilot study as you would for a large study. Once the sample size has been determined, then a percentage of the planned sample can be used for the pilot study. Use the statistical test rules of your study to set minimum participant numbers. For example, if a t-test is going to be used to find the mean difference in scores between your control and experimental groups (power of .80, $p < .05$, and effect size of .30) and the larger N = 174 in each group, then for the pilot you might consider using 20% of the sample, or 35 in each group; t-tests are robust with 30 units per group. Remember, too small of a pilot sample size may misguide the effect size that you are going to use for the larger study.

Writing the Sample Section of Your Proposal

Communication of the sampling plan is important when writing the sample section of your proposal. The sample is described within the proposal's Methods section. The Methods section usually begins with the study design, then the sample, followed by the procedures, instruments used, and types of analyses (Saver, 2011). The proposal reviewer is trying to determine if your proposal design and sampling method will have internal validity (the measured variable and not a confounding variable accounts for the results) and external validity (study results can be generalized to the population). If the study lacks validity, the findings might be erroneous; therefore, it is your responsibility to describe the planned sampling method, how the sampling frame will be designed, and how the estimated sample size was determined.

Therefore your write-up must provide the reader with sufficient information to make a judgment about your study's sampling decisions (Polit & Beck, 2008). The proposal section should include identifying the portion of the target population available to you for sampling (e.g., all patients seen at X facility). You should describe the study eligibility criteria (e.g., inclusion and exclusion criteria) and the planned sampling method (e.g., simple random sampling). If a power analysis was performed, the sample size and calculations should be clearly explained. And, finally, you should describe in sufficient detail the recruitment plan for the study participants.

Try It Now!

Determine the characteristics of the sample for this research question: Does an interactive video or one-on-one diabetic injection education improve self-injection among older adults on the medical-surgical unit? Identify the population, inclusion criteria, and exclusion criteria, as well as where you would obtain your sample.

References

DeMuth, J. E. (2008). Preparing for the first meeting with a statistician. *American Journal of Health-System Pharmacy, 65*(24), 2358–2366.

Gearing, R. E., Mian, I. A., Barber, J., & Ickowicz, A. (2006). A methodology for conducting retrospective chart review research in child and adolescent psychiatry. *Journal of the Canadian Academy of Child and Adolescent Psychiatry, 15*(3), 126–134.

Hedges, C., & Bliss-Holtz, J. (2006). Not too big, not too small, but just right: The dilemma of sample size estimation. *AACN Advanced Critical Care, 17*(3), 341–344.

Hoskins, C. N. & Mariano, C. (2004). Research in nursing and health: Understanding and using quantitative and qualitative methods (2nd ed.). Springer.

Polit, D. F., & Beck, C. T. (2008). *Nursing research: Generating and assessing evidence for nursing practice* (8th ed.). Philadelphia, PA: Lippincott, Williams, & Wilkins.

Sagan, C. Think Exist.com. Dr. Carl Sagan quotes (American Astronomer, Writer and Scientist, 1934-1996). Retrieved from http://thinkexist.com/quotation/somewhere-something_incredible_is_waiting_to_be/154069.html

Saver, C. (2011). *Anatomy of writing for publication for nurses*. Indianapolis, IN: Sigma Theta Tau International.

Yount, R. (2006). *Research design and statistical analysis for Christian ministry*. Retrieved from http://www.napce.org/

*"If the only tool you have is a hammer,
you tend to see every problem as a nail."*

–Abraham Maslow

Data Collection and Measurement

Christine Hedges

Now that you've chosen a research design (Chapter 7) and sample
(Chapter 8) for your study, you are probably anxious to begin collecting data. You collect data every day in patient care (vital signs,
lab results, intake and output) and you understand the importance
of clinical accuracy as you collect these clinical measures. You may
already be somewhat familiar with collecting other measures, or
metrics, for quality improvement (QI) purposes, such as collecting
information about falls, pressure ulcers, or patient satisfaction with
nursing care. You are also undoubtedly familiar with completing
surveys yourself.

But how do you start collecting data for a research study? And
is it any different from the types of data collection just described?
How do you select an instrument or a tool to collect data in a
research study? How can you be sure that most people will want to
complete your survey or fill out a questionnaire? This chapter helps
you understand some of the decisions that you must make *before*
selecting a "tool" or "instrument" (as measures are often called in
research), as well as things to consider when administering the
instrument and evaluating the results obtained from the measure.
This chapter discusses both instruments and the principles behind
measurement.

WHAT YOU'LL LEARN IN THIS CHAPTER

- Measurement, in research, is a way of assigning values to variables.

- There are many types of measures, and the choice of measure depends on the purpose of the study.

- Nurse researchers should strive to select measures that have established reliability and validity and that minimize error.

- Measurement tools are the property of individuals who developed them or groups who own the copyrights.

What Is a Measure?

Sometimes called a *tool* or *instrument* in quantitative research, a *measure* is simply a means of assigning a value, usually a number, to an item. Chapter 4 explains how to define variables and the difference between a *conceptual* and *operational* definition of the variables. Recall that the operational definition describes the method or instrument by which the variable will be measured, and it should be in agreement with the conceptual definition. A common mistake is measuring something similar to the variable of interest, but that is not quite the same thing.

For example, suppose you want to conduct a research study to determine if an intervention of quiet time and sleep-promotion activities results in improved sleep for the patients. How would you *measure* sleep? Because it is probably not practical to perform a full, objective polysomnography on each patient, you might opt for a cost effective paper-and-pencil, self-report questionnaire. Are you interested in how many *hours* of uninterrupted sleep the patient gets? You might consider having the patient complete a sleep diary in the morning following the intervention. If you are interested in whether the patient experiences less day-time *sleepiness* after the intervention, the Epworth Sleepiness Scale (Johns, 1991) is a measure to consider. If you are interested in the *quality* of the sleep, you might consider using the Pittsburgh Sleep Quality Index (PSQI) (Buysse, Reynolds, Monk, Berman, & Kupfer, 1989). But the PSQI includes the patient's sleep habits over the previous month before the hospitalization and is probably not the best choice for the purpose of evaluating this intervention. Sleep time, sleepiness, and habitual sleep quality are different concepts and should be measured or operationalized appropriately (Hedges, 2008).

Selecting a Measure: The Right Tool for the Right Job

One of the first questions you might ask is whether to measure with an instrument you have in hand (or can obtain easily), or whether to create or design a new instrument. To answer this question, let's look once again to our clinical practice.

If you want to measure your patient's blood pressure, there are options: You could measure it manually with an inflatable cuff and stethoscope, or you could use a blood pressure machine with an automatic cuff. If you work in the intensive care unit (ICU), your patient might even have an arterial line by which you could continuously monitor blood pressure. What do all of these methods have in common, and how do you know that the BP reading is accurate and trustworthy?

Well, you know to select an instrument (or tool) that is used to measure blood pressure. It needs to be in good working order, correctly calibrated and verified by the manufacturer, with appropriate safety and quality checks by your hospital. You would select an appropriate size cuff for your patient's arm circumference and correctly position the cuff on the upper arm with the bell of the stethoscope over the brachial artery before taking the reading. You are also aware that several factors can result in incorrect readings, such as wrapping the cuff too tightly or too loosely; faulty arm position; or deflating the cuff too quickly. You even know that an anxious patient can change the accuracy of the reading.

It is actually no different when selecting a tool or measure for your research purposes: You have a variety of tools from which to select; you should choose the correct one for your purpose; you should check that it is in good working order; and you should use it the way it was intended so that you can trust your results! Would you even consider creating your own blood pressure device and bringing it to work? Certainly not as long as there are accurate, tested, tried-and-true tools of the trade. Yet many nurses who are conducting their first clinical research study may attempt to create their own questionnaires rather than using an established, valid, and reliable measure. (There are times when no tool is available, but that topic is covered later in the chapter).

Q: *What is the difference between a questionnaire and a survey? Aren't they the same thing?*

A: *Survey* is the act of collecting the information; the questionnaire is the *form*. However, people sometimes use those terms interchangeably in everyday language.

The old adage *right tool for the right job* applies in research as much as it does in clinical practice. As suggested in the quote by Maslow (n.d.) at the beginning of this chapter, if you limit yourself to only one tool, survey, or measure that you know, you may become biased in your outlook or use the tool inappropriately. And in that case, you won't obtain results you can trust. Let's take a look at some of the types of data collection tools from which to choose and determine how you will know whether you can trust one.

Biophysiologic Measures

As a nurse, you are familiar with biophysiologic measures, such as blood pressure, temperature, and weight, that can be collected when clinical data is of interest to you. Because they are objective and usually available in the clinical setting, biophysiologic measures can be easy to use and often cost effective, as long as no new equipment needs to be purchased. However, biophysiologic measurement can become costly if new equipment needs to be purchased for your study. For instance, if you are studying workflow and want to measure distance walked by nurses, you might need to purchase pedometers that are not usually available on your unit, which adds cost to your study.

Observation

Another type of data collection is observation, often used to collect data about behaviors or personal characteristics such as hand hygiene or workplace communication patterns. Don't be fooled into thinking that observation is less costly, though. Keep in mind that observation involves time for a paid observer to watch and record, and then you have to pay for the transcription of observational data.

Self-Report

One of the first questions to be considered when collecting self-reports is whether you intend to collect numbers or words. If you are interested in a patient's subjective experience—in their own words—you will likely want to explore the collection of *qualitative* data. This can be in the form of focus groups, unstructured, semistructured, and structured individual interviews (see Chapter 12 for more information). If the participant's answers can be counted or quantified, you will be collecting quantitative data. Remember, you can ask questions about a how a subject *feels* and still quantify or put the response into numbers. For instance, pain or anxiety is a self-reported experience that can be reported qualitatively with words or quantitatively reported on a scale that assigns a number to the intensity.

Nurse researchers often survey research participants to collect self-reports. If you survey the participant face-to-face, you can assure that all data is completely collected, and you can settle discrepancies immediately. However, keep in mind that there is a loss of anonymity and a potential for bias when collecting the data in person. (Read Chapter 14 if you are fuzzy about the difference between anonymity and confidentiality.) Surveying face-to-face is useful with persons who may need more time and assistance—for example, when conducting research with frail elderly or pediatric participants—but the researcher must be cognizant of the special precautions needed with vulnerable populations (see Chapter 15 for more information).

Distributing questionnaires is favored by many clinical nurse researchers as they are self-administered (by the participants), are frequently inexpensive, and facilitate confidentiality or anonymity more readily. Let's look at some of the common types of self-report methods encountered in clinical research.

Questionnaires. Questionnaires are used to obtain information by paper and pencil or, more frequently now, by computer or online survey techniques (see Chapter 17 for more information). Questionnaires are considered a highly effective way to obtain responses in nursing and other types of behavioral research. One of the most frequent uses of the questionnaire format is collecting descriptive background or demographic information from your study participant. (Remember when I said that there were certain times that you would have to create your own tool? The demographic questionnaire is one you have to create!) Creating questionnaires takes skill and experience, and you should know some rules about questionnaire creation.

For instance, questions should be written at an appropriate reading level for the study participants. (A 6th or 8th grade reading level is usually preferred). You need to consider the length of the questionnaire, too. Although an 80-item questionnaire might easily be completed by a healthy nursing student, it is unlikely that your new postoperative cardiac surgical patient is going to have the energy and interest to complete such a questionnaire without becoming fatigued, and that's a fast path to ending up with incomplete data. Another guideline is that questionnaires should not ask for more than one response within the same question.

The following is an example of a poorly worded question:

1. How many hours of sleep do you get at night, and is it restful?

A better way to obtain this information is to use two questions:

1. How many hours of sleep do you usually get at night? _____

2. Do you feel rested upon awakening? Yes _____ No _____

In addition, questions should avoid forced responses. When creating a questionnaire, especially in the multiple-choice format, the responses should be mutually exclusive and collectively exhaustive. Put simply, that means there should not be more than one choice, and all available options should be in the response set. For example, you might ask nurses the following question:

What type of professional certification do you possess?

Your answer choices might be:

    a. Medical-surgical nursing

    b. Critical care nursing

    c. Emergency nursing

    d. Oncology nursing

    e. Perioperative nursing

Suppose the nurse was certified in *both* critical care and oncology? If only one response can be selected, the respondent is then forced to only choose one. Likewise, the nurse could be certified in behavioral health nursing, but it is not included in the list. Forcing the respondent to choose a response could result in meaningless data for the researcher.

Q: *Could I just add an answer choice labeled "Other"?*

A: Often adding a field labeled "Other" can help collect responses you may not have anticipated, but free-text responses make analysis more difficult because they may result in diverse responses that are not easily coded or categorized. It is best to carefully design the question to include as many possible choices so that "Other" is for rare or unusual responses only.

Finally, it's important to avoid questions that lead or bias the respondent. Consider this question and answer set:

If you are not professionally certified, when do you plan on taking the certification exam?

    a. Within the next 6 months

    b. Within one year

    c. Within the next 2 years

    d. Within the next 3 years

In this example, you are clearly suggesting your bias that taking a professional certification exam is desirable or expected.

Whether you are creating demographic questions or creating a questionnaire because no tool exists to elicit your topic of interest, it is important to have the items read by experts in your field and pilot tested in a small group as some problems are not uncovered until a trial is performed.

Scales. Scales are another form of self-report tool used in nursing and psychological research. Nurses often use them to elicit responses about attitudes, traits, or intensity of symptoms. You are probably already familiar with a variety of pain-rating scales in which a patient reports his or her pain intensity by choosing a number from 0 (no pain) to 10 (worst possible pain). See Figure 9.1.

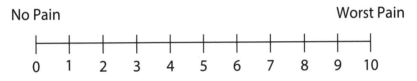

Figure 9.1   The 0–10 numeric pain rating scale

Another variation of this is a visual analog scale (VAS), which is used to quantify the intensity of subjective feelings such as pain or fatigue. In the VAS, a straight line, usually 100 mm, is labeled at either end and the respondent chooses the point on the line that corresponds to their experience. See Figure 9.2.

Likert scales are another type of attitude scale frequently seen in nursing, social science, and marketing research. Likert scales were originally developed to express levels of agreement or disagreement with statements, but the format has been extended to include frequency and evaluation of items. The Likert scale is typically comprised of a number of statements (called the *items*) with a number of balanced responses (typically five or seven) that correspond to levels of Agreement or Disagreement with the item. See Figure 9.3.

When the Likert scale has an odd number of responses, the neutral point is the midpoint. A Likert scale with an even number of responses (for example, four or six) doesn't have the neutral point, and there is argument whether or not this should be used as it may lead to a social desirability bias—you either have to agree or disagree to some extent (Dawes, 2008; Garland, 1991).

No Pain |

Worst Pain |

Figure 9.2   Visual analog scale (100 mm line)

Although there are advantages to self-report measures, there are also disadvantages that the researcher needs to keep in mind. A potential disadvantage of using attitude scales is referred to as *response set bias*. Put simply, this is the tendency for participants completing a self-report scale to do the following (Polit & Beck, 2010):

- Give the socially desirable response ("Yes, I floss every day!"), called the *social desirability response set bias*.

- Check off only the extreme highs or lows, such as strongly agree or strongly disagree ("I think everyone in my hospital is a team player!"), called the *extreme response set bias*.

- Consistently mark Agree or Disagree for all the questions regardless of the item (the yea-sayers and nay-sayers), known as the *acquiescence response set bias*.

Often researchers who develop scales using the Likert format use strategies to counterbalance negative and positive items (Polit and Beck, 2010). This is another reason to use a tool that is already developed—it's tried and true.

Directions: Indicate the degree to which you agree or disagree with the following statements:

1. Hand washing should be performed before entering a patient's room.

1	2	3	4	5
Strongly disagree	Disagree	Neither agree or disagree	Agree	Strongly agree

2. Hand hygiene should be performed even when gloves are used.

1	2	3	4	5
Strongly disagree	Disagree	Neither agree or disagree	Agree	Strongly agree

3. Nurses in my organization always perform hand hygiene.

1	2	3	4	5
Strongly disagree	Disagree	Neither agree or disagree	Agree	Strongly agree

Figure 9.3 Example of Likert scale items

There is also evidence that Likert scale responses may exhibit cultural differences. Researchers found cultural differences in Likert response patterns in one study of Chinese, Japanese, and Americans, including a greater tendency for Chinese and Japanese participants to choose a midpoint (neutral response) on positive emotions when compared to the American participants (Lee, Jones, Mineyama, & Zhang, 2002).

Measurement Concepts

Before you make any final decisions when choosing a tool or measure, you also need to consider some measurement concepts. This might sound a little scary, but it becomes very important when you get to the statistical analysis portion of your study.

Levels of Measurement

There are four hierarchal levels when thinking about measurement:

- Nominal

- Ordinal

- Interval

- Ratio

The lowest level of measurement is nominal (when you think nominal, think "name"). Variables described as nominal level can be named, categorized, and counted, but little else can be done statistically. Some examples of nominal-level data are items such as gender, religion, marital status, and occupation.

The next level of measurement is ordinal (think "order"). Like nominal variables, variables described as ordinal level can also be named, categorized, and counted, but they can also be put in some sort of order or hierarchy. Examples of ordinal level data are academic year in college (freshman, sophomore, junior, senior); functional status or ADL (independent, needs some assistance, needs total assistance); or level of agreement (strongly disagree, disagree, agree, strongly agree). Ordinal-level data is often referred to as "ranking" because there is a rank order of the items.

Both nominal and ordinal data are categorical, but take a look at the nominal-level measure "marital status." Can you say that being widowed is "higher" or "lower" than being single? Of course not! It wouldn't make sense. But look at the ordinal-level variable "year in college"; being a senior is a higher "rank" than being a sophomore.

Whereas nominal and ordinal are categorical data, interval and ratio represent continuous data and are considered higher levels of measurement. Interval-level data are items that have a rank order *and* there is an equal distance that can be measured between each item. (It sounds more sophisticated already!) Examples of interval-level data are systolic blood pressure in mmHg, IQ scores, and age. The highest level of data is ratio, and this can often seem confusing because it sounds so much like interval—in fact, many times interval and ratio are referred to together like this: *interval/ratio*. Ratio level data is only distinguished from interval in that it has a *meaningful or absolute zero*. For example, 0° Celsius could not be ratio level because it does not represent the absence of any temperature, since if we convert to Fahrenheit, it would be 32° F. But your savings account balance could be ratio as it could reach zero if you spent all the money in it.

The reason interval and ratio (continuous) data are higher level than nominal and ordinal (categorical) data is that interval/ratio can be reduced to a lower level, but the reverse is not possible (nominal and ordinal cannot be converted to interval ratio). Furthermore, greater statistical manipulations are possible. You can count and calculate percentages and frequencies, but you can also calculate means or averages. (The importance of the levels of measurement will become more evident as you read Chapter 11.)

Measurement Error

Another concept to consider is measurement error. In the natural world, and in the world of research, some amount of error exists. For example, each of us weighs a certain amount. When we step on a scale to weigh ourselves we see a number. This number may or may not be your actual weight. The difference between our actual or "real" weight and the number obtained on the measure (the scale) is the amount of error. Earlier we said that a blood pressure measurement could be affected by anything from an ill-fitting cuff to faulty equipment. Therefore, the patient's actual blood pressure may differ slightly from the one you obtain. This difference is the measurement error. Clearly you want to keep measurement error to a minimum with carefully selected tools.

Validity and Reliability

After you have chosen a tool or measure for your research study and have decided to use one that was developed by an expert (rather than create your own), how do you know if it is likely to give you accurate results? How do you know that *the expert's* tool is trustworthy? Can you be certain that it is precise and valid? Scales and questionnaires don't come with quality inspection labels, do they? Do you trust any measure or scale you find in a book or journal or online? You have to determine the validity and reliability of the tool.

Validity

What does it mean when you are asked to show a *valid* driver's license, or you have a restaurant coupon that says *valid* for 1 year? It implies that the license is authentic, or the coupon is acceptable, irrefutable for use. It's much the same with the validity of measurement tools. An instrument or tool is considered valid if it measures what it intends to measure. Returning to the example of measuring blood pressure, would you use a thermometer to measure blood pressure? Of course not! The thermometer is a good measurement tool that can give a valid reading of temperature, but it cannot give us a valid reading of blood pressure!

How do you know if your survey tool or questionnaire is valid? There are several ways you can assess an instrument's validity; you should consider these whenever you are selecting a tool for use in a research study. You should also keep validity in mind when you are appraising the tools used in a study you are reading when you're conducting an evidence-based practice (EBP) review. There are three broad categories or types of validity:

- **Content validity:** The instrument accurately measures the domain (or content) of the trait or concept.

- **Construct validity:** The degree to which the instrument measures the theoretical construct being studied.

- **Criterion-related validity:** How does it measure against a "gold standard" for that concept?

A research team investigated a new Critical-Care Pain Observation Tool (CPOT). They assessed the relationship between their new measure for pain and the "gold standard" of patient self-report of pain using advanced statistical techniques. This established the criterion validity of the CPOT (Gelinas, Fillion, Puntillo, Viens, & Fortier, 2006).

Establishing validity may not always involve advanced statistical procedures. Nurses who wish to establish content validity of a new questionnaire often use a "rudimentary" type of validity called *face validity* by asking experts to review the questions. For example, a nurse researcher wanted to develop a tool about nurses' attitudes toward pressure ulcer prevention. Once she had developed her questions, she asked three wound care nurses to assess the questions for content and accuracy using face validity (Russell-Babin, unpublished 2013).

Table 9.1 outlines the types of validity. When searching for a measure for your study, be sure to look for evidence that the measure has validity.

Table 9.1   Types of Instrument Validity

Category	Description	Examples
Content validity	Describes whether the instrument is accurately measuring the full domain (content) of a concept, characteristic, or trait	Content validity Face validity
Construct validity	Describes the degree to which the instrument measures the construct or trait	Convergent validity Discriminant validity

Category	Description	Examples
Criterion-related validity	Describes how the performance on a measure relates to the "gold standard," now or in the future	Concurrent validity Predictive validity

Adapted with permission from Hedges, C. (2008). What's in your toolbox? Considerations when selecting and evaluating instruments in clinical research. AACN Advanced Critical Care, 19(1), 19–22.

Reliability

Reliability refers to trustworthiness. In clinical practice, you gather data (vital signs, lab results) to make decisions about care. When you test your patient's blood sugar before administering insulin, you are depending on the reliability of the glucose meter results. You know that the results must be trustworthy in order for you to adjust the patient's dose based upon the results. Trustworthy or reliable results ensure that the findings are precise, stable, accurate, and dependable. If they were not, you could not practice with confidence! Here are some examples of types of reliability:

- Internal consistency reliability

- Test/retest (or *stability*) reliability

- Inter-rater (or *equivalence*) reliability

Internal consistency reliability. Internal consistency reliability, also referred to as *homogeneity*, describes a mechanism by which all of the items within an instrument capture the concept. One of the most common forms of internal consistency reliability calculated in nursing studies is the coefficient alpha, or *Cronbach's alpha*, which analyzes the items in a scale or questionnaire simultaneously to see the extent to which they reflect the phenomenon of interest. The Cronbach's alpha can range from .00 to + 1.00, whereby the higher the coefficient, the more reliable the measure. A good rule of thumb is to consider an instrument that has a Cronbach's alpha value of > .70 to have acceptable internal consistency reliability (Polit & Beck, 2010).

Test/retest reliability. Nurses often want to ensure that a particular measure is reliable if used on repeated administrations. A form of reliability that ensures that the measure works well or is stable on repeated administrations is known as *test/retest reliability*. Test/retest reliability only works with concepts considered to be fairly stable over time, such as self-esteem. It wouldn't work as well on a concept such as pain, which can change over time.

Inter-rater reliability. A third type of reliability ensures that the results of an instrument would provide equivalent results if performed by another person. This is known as inter-rater reliability. Returning to the example of the development of the CPOT, the investigator and another nurse researcher each completed the pain assessment, but were blinded to each other's results. They then compared their results statistically to calculate how closely their ratings reached agreement (Gelinas, et al., 2006). This can either be reported as a percent agreement by the two raters or a computation known as a Kappa (K) statistic. (Waltz, Strickland, & Lenz, 2010). If you are considering performing research to investigate a new tool in your clinical setting, one of the first steps should be to perform inter-rater reliability. Table 9.2 lists types of reliability.

Table 9.2   Types of Instrument Reliability

Type	Description	Examples
Internal consistency reliability (homogeneity)	Items within the instrument capture the concept	Split-half reliability Cronbach
Equivalence reliability	Instrument obtains the same or similar results as another measure or rater	Inter-rater reliability
Stability reliability	Instrument is consistent on repeated administrations	Test/retest reliability Alternate form reliability

Adapted with permission from Hedges, C. (2008). What's in your toolbox? Considerations when selecting and evaluating instruments in clinical research. AACN Advanced Critical Care, 19(1), 19–22.

Whether you are thinking of adopting a tool for your research study or evaluating the measurement section of a research study in EBP, you should look for evidence of both validity and reliability of the measures. This information is usually listed in the "Methods" section, right under "Instruments." When writing the "Methods" section of your own research proposal, be sure to support the instruments you intend to use with evidence of validity and reliability. In addition, you should describe each instrument and details about its administration, including approximately how long it will take to complete. Furthermore, you should use the instrument in its original form, without adding or deleting items. Otherwise, the instrument is no longer the original measure and the reliability and validly cannot be supported. It is essential that you obtain permission before copying, modifying, or using any existing tool, and you should give credit to the original developer (Waltz et al., 2010). Many instruments have short forms or brief versions available that have reliability and validity to support the altered version.

How to Locate Copies of Instruments for Research

There are several ways to find instruments and tools for use in research. By reading research studies or attending research conferences, you can learn what tools were used by other researchers that might be helpful for your study. Some journal articles are dedicated solely to the development of a tool or the comparison of several tools to address a particular phenomenon. Additionally, there are books, journals, and websites that are useful for locating instruments for use in research. Printed instruments are often protected by U.S. Copyright Law and the copyright can be held by either the author or a publishing company that charges for the use of the instrument and duplication of any scoring sheets. Therefore, it is imperative that you obtain permission to use or purchase the instrument. Frequently an author will generously grant you permission to use the instrument free of charge; in this case, you should keep a copy of the correspondence documenting permission in your research records. This correspondence is evidence of a legal transaction granting you permission to use the tool.

Q: *Our research team wants to study depression in postoperative cardiac surgical patients, but the tool we have found seems too long. Can't we just shorten it to two or three items?*

A: Respondent fatigue or burden related to a long tool is certainly a concern. But an instrument's reliability and validity were established on the tool in its complete form. Furthermore, it would be unethical to alter an instrument without permission from the developer of the instrument. Why don't you investigate to see if there is a short form (SF) or brief version of the instrument that has established reliability and validity? If it would make more sense to remove an item from the tool rather than create a new one, be sure to contact the developer of the tool for permission to remove an item. Remember that permission to use the tool is always expected, and reliability and validity of the new "altered tool" has not been established.

The science of developing instruments is a complex field of study and is often referred to as *psychometrics*. In fact, nurses who want to develop new instruments use a specialized research design known as *methodological research design*. Nurses who want to explore measurement issues in greater depth are referred to excellent resources such as *Measurement in Nursing and Health Research* by Waltz et al. (2010).

Try It Now!

Go back and find a research study that you read before. Look for evidence that the authors have discussed the properties of the tools/instruments used in the study. Is there evidence of *both* reliability and validity? Would you consider the instruments suitable for use in the study?

References

Buysse, D. J., Reynolds, C. F., Monk, T. H., Berman, S. R., Kupfer, D. J. (1989). The Pittsburgh Sleep Quality Index: A new instrument for psychiatric practice and research. *Psychiatry Research, 28*(2), 193–213.

Dawes, J. (2008). Do data characteristics change according to the number of scale points used? An experiment using 5 point, 7 point and 10 point scales. *International Journal of Market Research, 50*(1), 1–19.

Garland, R. (1991). The mid-point on a rating scale: Is it desirable? *Marketing Bulletin, 2,* 66–70.

Gelinas, C., Fillion, L., Puntillo, K. A., Viens, C., & Fortier, M. (2006). Validation of the Critical-Care Pain Observation Tool in adult patients. *American Journal of Critical Care, 15*(4), 420–427.

Hedges, C. (2008). What's in your toolbox? Considerations when selecting and evaluating instruments in clinical research. *AACN Advanced Critical Care, 19*(1), 19–22.

Johns, M. W. (1991). A new method for measuring daytime sleepiness: The Epworth Sleepiness Scale. *Sleep, 14*(6), 540–545.

Lee, J. W., Jones, P. S., Mineyama, Y., & Zhang, X. E. (2002). Cultural differences in responses to a Likert Scale. *Research in Nursing & Health, 25,* 295–306.

Maslow, A. (n.d). Retrieved September 25, 2013, from http://www.brainyquote.com/quotes/quotes/a/abrahammas126079.html

Polit D. F., & Beck, C. T. (2010). *Essentials of Nursing Research* (7th ed.). Philadelphia: Wolters Kluwer Health/Lippincott, Williams & Wilkins.

Russell-Babin, K. (2013). *A comparison of educational interventions to impact behavioral intent toward pressure ulcer prevention among nurses on medical surgical units* (Unpublished doctoral dissertation). Nova Southeastern University, Fort Lauderdale, FL.

Waltz, C., Strickland, O., & Lenz, E. (2010). *Measurement in Nursing and Health Research* (4th ed.). New York: Spring Publishing.

"The goal is to transform data into information, and information into insight."

–Carly Fiorina

Data Entry Basics

Noreen B. Brennan

10

The purpose of this chapter is to provide you with ideas of how to manage the data that you have collected. That process starts at the moment you have the idea to perform any type of research process, from a simple evaluation of a product to a doctoral dissertation. Two tools, the code book and data collection form, enable you to access and manipulate the data on a computer so that the research questions can be answered.

This chapter discusses creating data collection forms and tables for research, managing data, and identifying individuals who can provide help. It also identifies some of the common electronic tools and basic concepts of data entry. In addition, the chapter reviews data entry, keeping records and code books, securing data in password-protected computers, and writing the data entry section of a proposal.

The Literature Review

Let's say that you are interested in evaluating a new automated medication dispensing system. Where would you begin? The first step would be to review the current literature. As you have learned from the previous chapters, some of the questions that you would ask are:

- Has this been studied before? If so, what is known?

- What is known about this topic that may not have been considered?

WHAT YOU'LL LEARN IN THIS CHAPTER

- The code book and data collection form are essential tools for managing your data.

- Help with completing data entry for your study is available in many places, including working with biostatisticians, nurse scientists, and nursing informaticists.

- Choosing the right data analysis tool is an important part of your research study.

- Securing your data is essential and required by law.

- Is there already a valid and reliable tool to collect data about medication dispensing?

- What are the best search terms to use in this search?

- How can I narrow down the searched items?

- Is there an appropriate theoretical framework?

- In what settings has this research been done?

- How am I going to synthesize all of this information?

- What is or are my research questions/hypotheses?

As was suggested in Chapter 6, it is helpful to develop a table for research. Using our earlier example of the automated medication dispensing machine, set up a table that will help to summarize the literature review portion of your study (see Figure 10.1). You can change the column names to meet your needs, but column headings such as the following are usually a good place to start: Author, Year (study published), Sample, Instruments, Findings, and Limitations. Setting up your literature review in this format will help you to see at a glance what is known or unknown about a topic.

Author(s)	Year	Sample	Instruments	Findings	Limitations
Instruments Used					
Moran*	(2012)	150 RNs -42% M/S -58% ICU	Ease of Use (Foley, 2000); reliability and validity provided	M/S RNs found ADCs easier to use than did ICU RNs	Measured 2 units. Not representative of hospital population
Theoretical Framework					
Foley*	(2000)	None	None	Systems theory and Adult learning principles	Not research study, but provides framework for study

Fictitious studies

Figure 10.1   Example of literature review table

Creating Code Books and Data Collection Forms

There are many ways in which you can collect data for a statistical survey. The methods that are used to collect information from a sample of individuals have one main purpose: to collect the information in a systematic way. Over the last decade, there has been a shift in the modes used to collect data. The traditional paper-and-pencil interviewing (PAPI) has been replaced with computer-assisted interviewing (CAI). There has also been a shift from the traditional face-to-face surveys, telephone surveys, and mail surveys to web-based surveys (Bethlehem & Biffignandi, 2012). Whatever method of data collection you choose, you need to create two items to help manage the data: the code book and the data collection form.

 Are code books and data collection forms really necessary?

 Yes. The rationale for code books and data collection forms is to ensure the clear communication and understanding of the data that you have collected. They also provide a systematic way for you to analyze your data.

Code Books

The creation of a code book for your organization of data is important for a variety of reasons. The code book provides you with the definition of terms and codes used to summarize your data. It is also a good double-check to ensure that you have included all your variables. Lastly, it provides the "key" for the data values. You need to prepare the code book before you conduct your research. This is a great check to ensure that you have all your research questions.

Data coding is the translation of data into labeled categories suitable for computer processing. The code book is a dictionary listing names, labels, and code values in a data set (see Figure 10.2). For example, you may want to enter a variable that is a division of a group into two separate and distinct categories; these are known as dichotomous variables. For example, Yes and No are considered dichotomous variables, and you should enter them as numeric (i.e., 1 = Yes; 0 = No) data. This will make it easier when you do statistical analyses such as linear regression and descriptive statistics. Furthermore, it is easier to perform data entry using the keypad rather than Y = Yes and N = No.

Variable	Possible Values
ID	Values 1 to 200
Gender	1 = Male 2 = Female 99 = Missing
Unit	1 = Medical/Surgical 2 = ICU 99 = Missing
Ease of use of dispensing medication	1 = Easy to use 2 = Neutral (neither easy nor difficult) 3 = Difficult to use 99 = Missing
Education on automated dispensing machine	1 = Did not attend in-service or complete competency 2 = Attended in-service only 3 = Completed competency only 4 = Attended in-service and completed competency 99 = Missing
Highest level of education	1 = Diploma 2 = Associate degree 3 = Baccalaureate degree 4 = Master's degree 5 = Doctorate degree 99 = Missing

Figure 10.2   Example of a code book

Using our previous example of the automated dispensing machine, let's set up the initial coding of data:

1. Assign a unique identification number for each respondent. This is useful if you note a mistake in the data, as it enables you to backtrack to a unique respondent.

2. Decide what program you are using for your code book (i.e., Microsoft Word, Excel, or Access; or SPSS).

Q: *What is SPSS, and why would I need it?*

A: SPSS is an abbreviation for Statistical Product and Service Solutions (formerly Statistical Package for the Social Sciences). It is one of the most widely used software programs for statistical analysis in the social sciences.

3. Organize the code book for preparation for the data collection form.

4. Determine the data level (i.e., nominal, ordinal, interval, and ratio; see Chapter 9 for a review of levels of measurement). All responses, no matter what level of measurement, should be assigned numerical values so you can work with numerical data in the statistical programs.

5. Code all possible responses, including missing responses (in other words, places where the respondent has not given an answer) for each question.

The Benefits of Internet-Based Survey Tools

If you are using an Internet-based survey tool to collect responses, such as SurveyMonkey, you have the ability to download the results into a program like Microsoft Excel. For an extra fee in SurveyMonkey, you can have your data directly imported to a statistical software program such as SPSS. Many types of statistical analysis are available. In SPSS, computations such as: descriptive and bivariate analysis; inferential statistics (i.e., t-test, ANOVA, Chi-Square), and predictive models (i.e., linear regression and factor analysis) are available to assist with your data analysis.

Data Collection Forms

After you have created your code book, the next step is to create your data collection form. The data collection form is used to record scores and other information after your respondents have completed the survey instruments. The data collection form should be clear and easy to use. When constructing the data collection form, you should use unique descriptors for your column headings. For instance, if you are interested in querying respondents about Initial Nursing Education and Highest Level of Nursing Education you would not want to have two columns labeled Nursing Education. Having the two columns with the same name will cause confusion when you are ready to analyze your data.

Using the code book from Figure 10.2, construct a sample data collection form (see Figure 10.3). Here are some things to keep in mind as you construct your form:

- The form should be easy to understand.

- Each row should be specific to one respondent.

- Create the form in Excel or SPSS.

- Enter a unique ID number for each respondent.

- Include the date and time on the form.

- Print a hard copy and save the file in at least two locations.

Remember, the more systematic you are with preparing the collection of data the easier the rest of the process will be.

ID	Gender	Unit	Ease of Use	Education on ADM	Highest Education
001	1	2	2	1	2
002	2	1	3	1	3
003	2	99	3	3	3

Figure 10.3 Example of a data collection form

Basic Concepts of Data Entry

Here are several basic concepts that you need to know about good data entry:

- Before starting your study, think about the type of data needed to answer your question(s).

- Create clear, easy-to-use tables.

- If someone else is entering your data, make sure that they understand your data set. Take the time to teach the person how to enter the data from your data collection tool. You should also check their work.

- Always save your original data in a second area and medium, such as an external hard drive or password-protected and encrypted USB flash drive.

- Never delete the original data saved file.

- Perform data cleaning, which is the process of detecting and correcting or removing corrupt or inaccurate records from the table.

Knowing Where to Go for Help

Many individuals—biostatisticians, nurse scientists, and nursing informaticists—can assist you on your journey to completing data entry for your study. If you're in school, a great place to start is with your professor; or if are already practicing and doing research, work with someone who has experience conducting research. One of these individuals can serve as your mentor.

Biostatisticians

Many organizations utilize a biostatistician to analyze data for health care practitioners. A preliminary meeting with a biostatistician is a good starting point for preparing for the analysis of your data after you have completed your review of the literature. He or she may provide information regarding the type of statistical analysis that may or may not be possible given the nature of the tool you are planning to use and provide insight into how you can answer your research question. The biostatistician may see weaknesses in your tool or in your methodology that could prohibit answering your research questions. For example, you may want to know how the implementation of an automatic dispensing system affects nursing turnover; however, you do not have an instrument or tool to measure nursing turnover at your institution.

 How can the biostatistician help me plan my data collection?

 The biostatistician will help ensure that you have asked all of the necessary questions to address your areas of concern. For example, you may want to know how the implementation of an automatic medication dispensing system affects medication administration time; however, you do not have an instrument or tool to measure medication administration time at your institution. Without a question included at the beginning of your research, you have no data to address the medication administration time variable. The biostatistician will ensure that you have a measureable question in your instrument to evaluate medication administration time.

Nurse Scientists

Nurse scientists, if one is available in your organization, are another great resource as you develop your data entry tools for your research project. The nurse scientist role involves planning, implementing, and evaluating nursing research and other (EBP) activities.

Nursing Informaticists

For technical, computer, and Electronic Medical Records (EMR) help, you should seek out assistance from a nursing informaticist. According to the American Nurses Association, nurse informatics, "integrates nursing science, computer science, and information science to manage and communicate data, information, knowledge and wisdom in nursing practice" (ANA, 2013). Another resource is your organization's information technology (IT) department, especially when you have hardware or software issues. Often times, approval to add or delete certain software is under the purview of the organization because it needs to protect the integrity of its internal systems. Additionally, some programs require licenses for single or multiple users. Depending on the software packages purchased, licenses may be required for each individual user. Before you download software to any work computer, make sure that you review the organization's policies and procedures with regard to IT.

Online Courses

Perhaps you do not have all of these individuals available to you, so now what? There are a variety of online courses that might help expand your knowledge base. For example, various apps are available for your smartphone or tablet that provide free classes on software.

At no cost, you can download iTunes, which enables you to participate in an online course or listen to podcasts about different computer topics. Also, you can do an Internet search to find websites that will provide an introductory lesson on a variety of topics such as Microsoft Excel. Another free resource is YouTube, where you can find videos (and sometimes actual courses) on a variety of computer and research topics.

You can also check to see if there are classes, such as basic Microsoft Word and Excel, available at your organization or local community college. Some commercial computer stores, such as Microsoft and Apple, also offer an array of classes to their customers (some are fee based).

Getting Acquainted with Key Software

There are certain programs we suggest you become familiar with, including a word-processing program such as Microsoft Word, a statistical program such as Microsoft Excel, and presentation software such as Microsoft PowerPoint. Companies other than Microsoft also offer programs for word processing, statistics, and presentations; it is really your preference of what you're most comfortable using. Becoming familiar with such programs will help you organize your literature review, assist with setting up your spreadsheets for calculations, and help you create your manuscript and presentation.

For example, word-processing programs have robust thesaurus, spelling, and grammar check features. For your data analysis, there are many computing programs, including Excel, SPSS, and Statistical Analysis System (SAS). These programs vary in terms of complexity and applicability. For example, Excel can be used to store data that you have entered or downloaded from another program. In addition, with Excel you can download add-ins that will do statistical analyses. A word of caution, no matter which computer software program you use: Please remember that if you put garbage in, you will get garbage out.

Help with Statistical Analysis Software

This website from IBM is useful for finding out further information on statistical software: http://www-01.ibm.com/software/analytics/spss/

As already mentioned, SPSS is the most widely used program for statistical analysis in the social sciences. This software package enables you to perform descriptive, bivariate, nonparametric tests, and parametric statistics. If you are a student you can purchase the grad pack, which enables you to perform many of the statistical analyses at a reasonable cost. SAS, another available statistical program, is more complex and requires programming language knowledge.

Q: *Do I need to purchase a statistical software program before beginning the research study?*

A: That depends on a number of considerations. If you are doing very basic descriptive statistical analysis, then you should be fine with a program like Excel. If you are comfortable with Excel, then we suggest getting the add-in statistical package. SPSS has a format similar to Excel; it is set up as a worksheet. However, the difference is that the cells in SPSS do not have the capability of doing math functions. You can download or import your Excel spreadsheets easily into SPSS.

Before you buy any program, find out if your organization or school has programs available for your use. If you are a student, you can purchase the grad package of SPSS for about $100. This might be a wise investment if you are going to be doing many research studies because SPSS can perform more functions than Excel.

Securing Your Data

You have probably heard the story about data security, with a little variation, that goes something like this:

> "Did you hear what happened to Frank?"
>
> "No, do tell!"
>
> "Well in order to catch up on some work, Frank downloaded the research study onto his USB memory stick and took the information home—you know, dates of birth, Social Security numbers, etc.—all that personal information, and now Frank can't locate the memory stick. Of course, it was not encrypted or password protected. The file had more than 500 subjects' information."
>
> "Frank is in some serious trouble."

Many times, we hear this same story about data, whether at work, school, or through media reports. Whether the story involves use of a memory stick/USB drive/jump drive which is unprotected, a laptop that is not password protected, or a computer that is left with the last user logged on, a security breach is likely to happen. Securing of data is extremely important in all aspects of data collection, retention, and storage. All data should be securely stored to prevent unauthorized access, disclosure, or loss.

Data security is so important that there are laws regarding protection and storage of information. The Health Insurance Portability and Accountability Act of 1996 (HIPAA) includes the Security Rule, which establishes national standards to protect individuals' electronic personal health information. HIPAA-covered entities and their business associates must provide notification following a breach of unsecured protected health information. This is required by section 13402(e)(4) of the Health Information Technology for Economic and Clinical Health (HITECH) Act. Breaches of unsecured protected health information affecting 500 or more individuals are posted online (http://www.hhs.gov). In the reported cases, most often a computer or jump drive is reported stolen. Many organizations will not permit the use of unsecured jump drives and as such have introduced encrypted jump drives, which require a username and password in order to access the data or information on the external drive.

Q: *Do I really need to have my data secured?*

A: Yes. Yes. Yes. Even if you are not using Protected Health Information (PHI) or personal demographic data of your respondents, you want to get into the habit of using password-protected computers and external hard drives. In fact, when you submit your proposals of research to the Institutional Review Board (IRB), you will be responsible for addressing how you plan to keep your data secure.

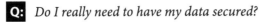

More About HIPAA Regulations

You can find the official website of the Department of Health and Human Services (HHS) at www.HHS.gov. The purpose of the website is to protect the health of all Americans and provide information regarding HIPAA regulations.

Institution Review Boards (IRBs) require investigators to provide information, which describes the mechanisms used to secure data obtained in the study. Security measures for your research should be appropriate to the degree of risk in the study and should be part of your research plan. You should address the following points:

- Where all personal data—whether recorded on paper, audio, video, or computer—will be stored

- The security procedures you will take for storing and transporting physical data

- The arrangements in place to prevent theft of data

- How access to data will be restricted

- Password-protection procedures used to protect electronic data

- Security arrangements if data are processed off-site

- How data will be disposed of at the end of the study

IRBs review computer and Internet-based research protocols using the same considerations and standards of approval of research as noncomputer-based studies. (For more on this topic, please see Chapter 17.)

Lastly, to avoid the liabilities associated with the loss or compromise of data and devices, there are some safeguards you should take:

- Assign Unique ID numbers for all respondents instead of using names.

- Ensure that laptops are password protected.

- Ensure that external USB data storage devices are password protected and encoded.

- If using websites such as SurveyMonkey for data collection, review their security settings (look for data encryption).

- Ensure your computer has the most up-to-date firewalls and virus protection.

- Review your organization's Security Policies and Procedures (i.e. HIPAA).

In summary, securing your data and devices should be a top priority when you are embarking on collecting and storing data. As investigators, we are responsible for describing and following through on the plans for securing our data. We should employ the tools and technologies that are available to help us ensure security.

Writing the Data Collection Section of Your Proposal

In writing the "Data Collection" section of your proposal, you describe how you will collect and protect your data. You should include the data you will be collecting, how it will be collected (online, paper and pencil, etc.), and where the data will be stored. IRBs are particularly interested in how you will secure and protect the data. For example, you should say that your electronic data will be secured on a password-protected computer. If you have collected data with pencil and paper, you should say that it will be secured in a locked filing cabinet in a locked office and note the location of the office, whether it is at home or work. Also, you must include who, in addition to the principal investigator, will have access to the data. All of this information may be included in the procedure section of the proposal under "Methods."

Try It Now!

You are leading a research study that is investigating the effects of gender differences on reports of experiences of workplace aggression (Scale 1= Never; 2= Daily; 3= Weekly; 4 = Monthly). From your literature review you have learned that years working in nursing, education preparation, race, and unit type are important variables. You will be collecting data from nurses working in the three hospitals in your health care network. Design a data collection form and code book that address the following variables:

- Gender

- Hospital

- Years in Nursing

- Educational Preparation

- Race

- Unit Type

References

American Nurses Association. (2013). Revised Nursing Informatics: Practice Scope and Standards of Practice. Retrieved from http://www.nursingworld.org/HomepageCategory/NursingInsider/ Archive_1/2008NI/Jan08NI/RevisedNursingInformaticsPracticeScopeandStandardsofPractice.aspx

Bethlehem, J., & Biffignandi, S. (2012). *Handbook of web surveys: Wiley handbooks in survey methodology* (pp. 567). New Jersey: John Wiley & Sons.

*"If the statistics are boring,
then you've got the wrong numbers."*

–Edward Tufte

Analyzing Your Findings

Elizabeth Heavey

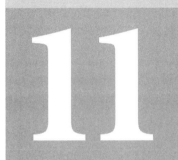

Nurses immersed in clinical practice frequently have excellent ideas about what is and is not working for their patients. They note commonalities and differences in how patients respond to treatment, similarities among patients admitted with the same diagnosis, and differences among those who do well and those who do not do well. These keen observations are a critical starting point to developing a research idea or hypothesis.

Unfortunately, many nurses are not confident in their abilities to understand or apply statistical techniques, which limits the development of nursing research. It also limits patient care because these great ideas frequently do not get developed or explored until someone in another profession picks up the interest. Nurses are on the frontline of day-to-day patient care. It can take a long time before members of other professions recognize some of the critical observations we make early on. This chapter covers basic concepts in statistical analysis, statistical versus clinical significance, common descriptive and inferential statistics utilized in nursing research, and preparation of the "Analysis" section of a research proposal.

WHAT YOU'LL LEARN IN THIS CHAPTER

- In statistics, conclusions are always voiced in terms of probability, not certainty.

- In order to establish *clinical significance*, you must establish *statistical significance*.

- It is a wise idea to obtain a statistical consultation early in your research study to ensure the project direction will lend itself to the type of analysis you would like to do.

Understanding the Meaning of Probability

The reality of life and the reality of statistics are that our conclusions are always voiced in terms of probability rather than certainty. Sometimes we are right, and sometimes we are wrong.

For example, if you are working on your unit and a stable postsurgical patient reports feeling like he might have torn his abdominal incision sutures when he moved, you don't immediately notify the surgeon of record. You continue to assess the patient and collect observations until you are more certain whether the patient is experiencing normal post-surgical pain or whether wound dehiscence is a significant concern.

Depending on the situation and the ramifications of being incorrect, you might need only a small number of observations before you conclude that there is a significant concern. This would be the case if you pull back the sheets and realize his gown and surgical dressing are soaked in blood while his blood pressure is dropping rapidly. In this situation you call the surgeon immediately.

If a situation appears to be as you expect—the patient is stable and the ramifications of prematurely alerting the surgeon are a concern—you may collect a larger number of observations before determining if what you are seeing is significantly different from what you expect in a safe situation. You might do this if you assess the patient and his vital signs are stable, he is in no apparent distress, and his surgical dressing is dry and intact. You would probably give him his prn pain medication and continue to monitor the situation. The danger in doing so is that while you are making the observations to develop a higher level of certainty, you might lose critical time waiting to be more certain. Nurses have to make these types of decisions on a regular basis, so most of us understand probability already.

From this example you can see what we mean about conclusions being in terms of probability rather than certainty. Nurses can use statistics to determine if what we see is significantly different or significantly associated before we draw a conclusion. We want to be reasonably certain, but we also don't want to wait too long trying to establish more certainty than we might reasonably need. As researchers, we establish the level of certainty we need to reach based on the present situation and the ramifications of being wrong. We then collect a sufficiently large number of observations to support the difference or association we think is present, and we test the data using statistics to determine the significance level that is reached.

Explaining Statistical Significance in Nonstatistical Language

The question you, as a researcher, should ask anytime you begin to determine if there is a statistically significant difference is fairly basic: Is what you are seeing different enough from what you would expect to see that you should be concerned and recommend a change?

For example, if your plan is to medicate a patient for pain, and you notice that the patient is bleeding through a wound dehiscence, you need to change your plan from delivering routine pain medication to obtaining immediate assistance. In the absence of evidence that the pain is anything other than normal postoperative pain, you can maintain your original expectation and medicate as ordered.

You make these decisions after collecting your data and analyzing it. If you find a statistically significant result, then you have found a difference that—if it's also clinically important—directs a change in the course of action. If you do not find a statistically significant result, then you do not find a difference, and you have no reason to change your current approach.

Additional Sources for Understanding Statistical Information

For an introductory discussion of the specific tests as well as other important concepts mentioned in this chapter, please see *Statistics for Nursing, A Practical Approach*, 2nd Edition by E. Heavey (2013).

For a graduate-level statistics book, we recommend the following:

- *Statistical Methods for Health Care Research*, 5th Edition by B. Munro (2005)
- *Statistics and Data Analysis for Nursing Research*, 2nd Edition by D. Polit (2010)

Getting a Statistical Consultation

I have a big secret that I share with nurses who have ideas and are intimidated by having to do analysis: Doing analysis isn't really that bad! Running a code; maintaining the safety and care of 12 patients per shift; helping a family say goodbye to a dying loved one; getting up and going to work after you've had the flu for a week and your kids are still sick and your laundry pile is huge—those things are much, much harder than doing some basic statistics! The real key is knowing what you know, being confident that what you know is valuable, and knowing where you need some help and guidance.

For example, I would be out of my league working in an adult surgical Intensive Care Unit (ICU). (I am a nurse-midwife and my only critical care experience is in the neonatal ICU.) But if for some reason I had to work in an ICU, I would certainly find some preceptors who know what they are doing and seek their advice, direction, and—in the beginning—their direct supervision. Statistics is no different from working on a unit with which you're not familiar. You have the idea; now get some help. You might be surprised at how much you can do with some friendly assistance. After some time you will build and develop additional skills that make it less intimidating to tackle future projects.

For any beginning nurse researcher, statistical consultation is a critical part of the research study. It is a wise idea to obtain a statistical consultation early in the project to ensure the project direction will lend itself to the type of analysis you would like to do. In addition, a consultation after the data is collected is wise to ensure that you have completed an appropriate analysis and have interpreted it correctly.

Statistical consultation is available from many sources. If you work in a hospital or are associated with a university that has nurse scientists or clinical nurse researchers, start by talking with those people. Nurses trained in statistics are frequently the individuals other nurses most easily understand, and they also relate well to the limitations and opportunities your specific clinical site may have.

Q: *Is there anything special I need to consider when deciding to work with a statistical consultant?*

A: It is very important that you work with a consultant who is willing and able to explain their recommendations to you and someone with whom you are comfortable asking the basic questions that beginning nurse researchers typically have. In any case, select someone who has the time, availability, and expertise you need. More importantly, you should find someone you can work with well for a period of time. Research studies are rarely short and can require a great deal of communication.

In some cases, the statistician completes the analysis as well, but it is still critical for you to understand what type of analysis is being done and why it is being done. You also need to understand any limitations the analysis may create in the interpretation of the data. The rest of this chapter is meant to help you with these things. This chapter won't necessarily teach you to tackle the statistics on your own, but it will help you have a reasonably educated discussion with a statistical consultant and help you understand what that consultant may recommend.

Q: *Our research team wants to collect data and then consult with a statistician to analyze the results. Why is it important to consult with the statistician before beginning the study rather than waiting until after we have collected our data?*

A: There is a quote by the famous statistician R.A. Fisher that says: "To consult the statistician after an experiment is finished is often merely to ask him to conduct a *post mortem* examination. He can perhaps say what the experiment died of" (Presidential Address to the First Indian Statistical Congress, 1938). When you consult with your statistician before you begin your research, that person can help you with sample size estimation, design decisions that will affect data collection, and even setting up your code book or data collection tools. It is never wise to ask someone to try to make sense of data that has been collected inappropriately. Unless you are a very experienced researcher, seek help first!

The Research Question

As you begin your research, we can't overemphasize the importance of understanding the question you are asking. This idea might seem very basic, but, as mentioned previously in the book, it is essential to develop your research question with thought and precision as it will be used to direct the data collection and analysis.

After you've determined your question, you should consider what sources of data may already exist that might answer the question, which saves you a lot of time and energy that you would otherwise expend in collecting data. When you establish what type of data you have or will collect, you need to examine the variables you have and establish the level of measurement for each. This affects the type of statistical analysis you will be able to perform (see Chapter 9 for a review of levels of measurement). Look at any variables that are not at the interval/ratio level and make sure you are either collecting them at the highest level possible or have a good reason not to do so.

For example, if you have a variable such as total cholesterol and you plan to record the measure as "high" or "low," you are collecting the data at a nominal level only. However, if you record the actual serum cholesterol reading, then you have reached the interval level and can perform more robust statistical analysis involving this variable. Perhaps you don't anticipate the cholesterol level being terribly important in your research, and the data is already available in the nominal form; in that case, you might decide it is not worth the additional time and financial cost associated with collecting the variable at a higher level of measurement. That is okay as long as you have thought it through. If you think total cholesterol may be a critical variable, you might want to collect the variable at a higher level of measurement. Then you can choose to recode the total serum cholesterol as "high" and "low" after collecting the actual number if it is helpful for your research. However, if you collect the data at the nominal level only, then you cannot recode it into interval/ratio level data.

Hypothesis Testing

As you learned in Chapter 4, the null hypothesis (null=no) is phrased as a lack of relationship, association, or difference between the independent and dependent variables. The alternative hypothesis is the existence of a relationship or difference among the independent and dependent variables. The alternative hypothesis is usually what the researcher believes the study will show. For example, if you think there is a relationship between total serum cholesterol (independent variable) and systolic blood pressure (dependent variable) and want to perform a study, then you may include the following hypotheses:

> **Null Hypothesis (H_0):** There is no association between total serum cholesterol and systolic blood pressure.

> **Alternative Hypothesis (H_1):** Higher serum cholesterol is associated with higher systolic blood pressure. (Or, if you prefer to use a nondirectional alternative hypothesis you may use the following: Serum cholesterol is associated with systolic blood pressure.)

How to Determine Statistical Significance

By now you have a clear research question, you've developed your hypotheses, and you have an understanding of your variables and how you will measure them. You are actually ready for an initial interaction with a statistical consultant. Your statistical consultant can help you determine the level of certainty you want to set for your conclusion, which will be used to determine whether any association or difference you find is significant.

After determining these factors, you would then examine the data analysis for a test statistic (result from the analysis) and the corresponding probability of this result (p value) to determine if you have a statistically significant result. If the probability, or p value, is less than alpha, you would reject the null hypothesis. Your results are then said to support the alternative hypothesis. If you do not have statistically significant results ($p >$ alpha), then you would fail to reject the null and conclude there is no relationship, association, or difference between the variables.

Both of the selected levels of alpha and power, combined with the size of the difference or association, help determine what size sample you need to collect. Determining the appropriate sample size can be a complicated but critical step in ensuring your research reaches the correct conclusion. It is a good idea to involve a statistical consultant in this step early in the study. (See Chapter 8 for a review of sample size.)

Types of Statistics

Most research studies involve the use of descriptive and inferential statistics, which are distinctly different types of measurements. Descriptive statistics are just what they sound like. They are measures that describe the sample or population with which you are working. You can use descriptive statistics to present or summarize actual data, and they are also helpful in identifying patterns or comparing samples to a population. However, descriptive statistics are limited to being helpful information about the sample that is actually measured. You should not generalize them to a population. You can, however, use them to compare a sample to the population from which it is drawn and illustrate that the sample is representative of the original population.

For example, if the population that interests you is registered nurses in New York State and you know that 80% of the registered nurses in New York are female, a representative sample of nurses collected in your study should also be approximately 80% female. If the sample is instead 40% female, then you did not collect a representative sample, which limits your ability to generalize your results to the population of interest. We will come back to this point a little later in the chapter. First, let's take a look at the two different kinds of statistics that are frequently used in nursing research.

Descriptive Statistics

Descriptive statistics include the frequency of the observations; the measures of central tendency, or the "center" of the variable's measurements, such as the mean, the median, and the mode; and the measures of the spread of the sample, such as range and standard deviation. We can also look for associations between variables in one sample using descriptive statistics and a process called *correlation*.

Frequency of observations. The frequency of the observations for each independent variable is usually presented in the beginning of the study. For example, in the study of 200 New York State nurses, you might think that the gender and age of the nurse, as well as the shift worked, affects the dependent variable of job satisfaction. In this case, you might include a table (see Table 11.1) that includes the absolute number of nurses in each category of your independent variables (n) as well as what percent of the sample these observations are (%).

Table 11.1   New York State Nurses Sample

Independent Variable	n (%)
Male	20 (10%)
Female	180 (90%)
20–30 years	60 (30%)
31–40 years	80 (40%)
41 years and older	60 (30%)
Days	150 (75%)
Nights	50 (25%)

These types of tables enable the readers of your research to get a good idea of what your sample includes or may be missing. For example, in the preceding table you don't tell the reader how you may have categorized nurses who work straight evenings, which may be problematic. Tables are a quick and easy way to get your main points across in any research article.

Central tendency. If you want to describe your sample further, you may include measures of central tendency, which describe how the values of a variable cluster. The measure of central tendency you can report depends on the level of measurement for the variable (see Table 11.2).

Table 11.2   Measures of Central Tendency

Measure of Central Tendency	Definition	Level of Measurement required
Mean	The "average" or the sum of the variables divided by the number of observations	Requires interval or ratio level data; cannot be determined for ordinal or nominal variables
Median	After lining up the values of all the observations from least to most, the value in the middle (with an even number of observations, the median is the average of the two central observations)	Requires ordinal-, interval-, or ratio-level data; cannot be determined for nominal-level variables
Mode	The most frequently occurring value or category	Can be determined with all levels of variables, including nominal

Again using the New York State nurses example, you cannot report the mean or average gender in your sample because gender is measured at a nominal level. But you can report the mode for the gender variable in this study, which would be female. If you gather the age information at an interval/ratio level (each nurse's actual age), before you put it in the categories in the table, you can report a mean age in your sample, which may be 38 years old. However, if you collect the age data in the categories listed previously, you are able to report the mode and median, which would both be 31–40 years old. The measure of central tendency you find useful depends on both the level of measurement and the current situation. (For further discussion of the situations in which you might prefer one over the other, please see Chapter 3 in Heavey [2013], *Statistics for Nursing: A Practical Approach*, 2nd Edition.)

Spread of the sample. When you describe your sample, you may also want to include measures that tell the reader how close the observations were to the middle in the relevant variables. For example, you may know that the mean or average age in your sample is 38, but a sample that is mostly made up of nurses who are close to the age of 38 may be associated with different results from one in which there are many nurses who are younger than 38 and older than 38. The *range* of the variable simply tells you the difference between the maximum and minimum values. The *standard deviation* takes this idea one step further and tells you the average distance the values are from the variable's center.

In this example, the sample in which most of the nurses are close to 38 years old might have a standard deviation of 1 (which means most of the nurses in your sample are about one year older or younger than your mean of 38). The sample in which there are many younger and older nurses may still have the same mean of 38, but the standard deviation might be 10, indicating that on average the nurses ages are 10 years older or younger than the mean age. The sample with the larger standard deviation has a larger variance in ages in the group. This information might impact your interpretation of the data and is frequently useful.

Correlation. Another commonly used descriptive statistic is the various forms of correlation. *Correlations* look for the association between two variables in one sample and can be measured by direction and strength. A *positive correlation* has a positive value and means the values of both variables move together in the same direction. For example, height and weight are generally positively correlated. As height increases, weight increases as well; and when height decreases, weight decreases (even though they are both decreasing, they are still moving in the same direction, which is a positive correlation). A *negative correlation* is said to occur when the two variables move in opposite directions. For example, there is a negative correlation between hours of sleep and a nurse's fatigue. The more sleep a nurse has, the less fatigue he/she will generally experience, and vice versa.

The strength of the correlation is reflected in the value of the *correlation coefficient*, which can range from –1 to +1. A correlation coefficient of –1 is a strong negative correlation, and a correlation coefficient of +1 is a strong positive correlation. The type of correlation you can use in your study is determined by examining the levels of measurement for each of the variables you want to correlate. Note in Table 11.3 that the variable that has the lowest level of measurement is what is used to determine what correlation coefficient you should report. For example, if you want to determine the correlation between a nominal-level variable and a ratio-level variable, you must complete the Chi-Square test because the nominal-level variable drives the decision for which correlation is appropriate. (More information is available about the Chi-Square test in the Inferential Statistics section of this chapter.)

Table 11.3   Correlation Coefficients for Variables Collected in one Independent Sample (No Comparison Group)

Lowest Level of Variable Involved in the Correlation	Appropriate Correlation and Test Statistic	Clinical Example
Nominal	Chi-Square (χ^2)	Is there an association between shift worked and marital status among nurses at my hospital?
Ordinal	Spearman's Correlation (or rho)	Is there an association between heart rate (HR) and pain in hospitalized children? (HR measured as beats per minute; pain measured as mild/moderate/severe)
Interval/ratio	Pearson's Correlation (r)	Is there an association between heart rate and blood pressure among men attending an Alcoholics Anonymous meeting?

These tests simply look for associations or relationships, not differences between groups. For example, in a sample of nurses working extended shifts, a relationship was found between hours worked and the number of medication errors.
Reprinted with permission from Heavey (2013), Statistics for Nursing: A Practical Approach, *2nd Edition, Jones & Bartlett.*

Inferential Statistics

After you have finished using statistics to describe your data, you will want to proceed to the use of inferential statistics. *Inferential statistics* uses your sample data to estimate and draw a conclusion about the population from which it was drawn. Remember these types of conclusions are always probabilities—never certainties—and you must consider the possibility of error. Nursing research frequently utilizes the inferential analyses included in Tables 11.4 and 11.5. You will see that the type of question you are asking, the type of sample you have collected, and the level of measurement affect the decision of what test to use in that particular situation.

Chi-Square test. The Chi-Square test looks for a difference or association in two or more independent samples when the outcome variable is at the nominal or ordinal level. For example, if you measure the highest level of nursing education as ADN, BSN, MS, PhD and want to determine if there is a difference in the level of nursing education achieved (dependent variable) for male and female nurses (independent variable), the Chi-Square test might be appropriate and will produce a χ^2 test statistic with a corresponding p value.

McNemar's test. If instead you had a nominal or ordinal outcome variable but had two dependent samples, such as the driver and passenger in the same car involved in a car accident, you may use a McNemars test, which is similar to a Chi-Square test but accommodates the dependency of the samples. This test produces a McNemars test statistic χ^2 and a corresponding p value.

Student t-test. The student t-test is used to determine if there is a difference in the average value of a variable in two independent samples when the outcome variable is at the interval or ratio level. For example, do Asian Americans have higher mean total cholesterol (dependent variable) than African Americans? You can use this same test to compare differences in the mean in an outcome variable at the interval/ratio level among dependent samples. It just requires one to use the t-test table values that accommodate dependent samples. The student t-test produces a t statistic, which has a corresponding p value.

ANOVA test. When looking for a difference in the mean value of an outcome variable at the interval/ratio level among more than two groups, a researcher might consider an Analysis of Variance (ANOVA) test, which produces an F statistic with a corresponding p value. The ANOVA test compares the differences between the groups (numerator) to the differences within the groups (denominator). The larger the differences are between the groups compared to the differences within the groups, the larger the F value. However, even a large F value still has a corresponding p value that is used to determine the statistical significance of the test.

Q: *When the test statistics are reported, what should I look for?*

A: These techniques involve testing your data to look for a significant difference or association. Applying these tests produces a result called a test statistic. The test statistic depends on what test is utilized. Each test statistic has a corresponding probability, or p value. So, no matter what the test statistic is, it is essential to examine the corresponding p value to determine if there is statistical significance. For example, if your study utilizes an alpha of 0.05 and the result includes an F statistic with a p value of 0.03, the p value is less than the alpha, so the results are statistically significant. If, however, your study uses a t-test and reports a p value of 0.13, the p value is greater than the alpha, so you know there is not a significant difference or association between the variables being examined.

A specialized form of ANOVA called *Repeat Measure ANOVA* can also be used to examine the differences in an outcome variable at the interval/ratio level among one group with the outcome variable measured at multiple points over time. For example, the researcher may use this approach to determine if there is an improvement in the general knowledge score for a group given a pretest, an intervention, and then a 6-week posttest and a 12-week posttest. There will again be an *F* statistic with a corresponding *p* value.

Table 11.4 Tests That Look for Differences or Compare at Least Two Groups or Samples

Sample Type	Level of Dependent or Outcome Variable	Test and Test Statistic	Research Example
Two independent samples	Nominal or Ordinal	Chi-Square (χ^2 and corresponding probability or *p* value)	Is there a difference in the level of nursing education achieved for male and female nurses? (Independent variable is nominal–male/female, dependent variable is ordinal with four levels-ADN, BSN, MS, PhD,)
Two dependent samples	Nominal or Ordinal	McNemar's (χ^2 and corresponding probability or *p* value)	In motor vehicle accidents involving a passenger and a driver, is the driver or the passenger more likely to experience a head injury? (Independent variable of driver/passenger are related because they are in the same car and therefore create two dependent samples; dependent variable head injury is yes/no or nominal)
Two independent samples	Interval/Ratio	T-test for independent samples (*t* and corresponding probability or *p* value)	Do Asian Americans have a higher mean total cholesterol than African Americans in a random sample of 10,000 Florida state residents? (Independent variable which creates the two independent samples is race; dependent variable mean total cholesterol is interval/ratio)

continues

Table 11.4   Tests That Look for Differences or Compare at Least Two Groups or Samples   *continued*

Sample Type	Level of Dependent or Outcome Variable	Test and Test Statistic	Research Example
Two dependent samples	Interval/Ratio	T-test for dependent samples (*t* and corresponding probability or *p* value)	Do husbands and wives have a difference in their mean total cholesterol? (Independent variable husband/wife creates two dependent samples because they are related with the dependent variable of mean total cholesterol, which is interval/ratio)
Two or more groups or samples	Interval/Ratio	Analysis of Variance (ANOVA) (*F* and corresponding probability or *p* value)	Is there a difference in the mean body mass index among nurses who work days, evenings, or nights? (The independent variable creates three independent samples to compare –shift worked, with a dependent variable of BMI at the interval/ratio level)
One group with outcomes measured at multiple points over time	Interval/Ratio	Repeat Measures ANOVA (*F* and corresponding probability or *p* value)	Is there an improvement in a general knowledge score for a sixth grade class given a pretest, then an educational intervention followed by a 6-week posttest, and a 12-week posttest? (Only one group with the dependent variable or outcome of an interval/ratio test score at multiple points over time).

Note: Samples or groups can be created by the levels of the independent variable. For example, gender may be your independent variable and the groups you are interested in comparing are men and women creating two samples. Table reprinted with permission from Heavey, E. (2013). Statistics for Nursing: A Practical Approach, *2nd Edition, Jones and Bartlett.*

Regression. Additional analysis options many researchers choose to use involve the techniques of multiple and logistic regression. These options allow the researcher to examine the effect of multiple independent variables on a single dependent variable (see Table 11.5). For example, if the researcher believes that maternal age and smoking both impact infant birth weight, the relationship between maternal age and infant birth weight can be seen while controlling for the impact of smoking on infant birth weight. Both techniques produce a variety of values that must be interpreted in conjunction with one another to build or develop the best statistical model. Beginning researchers would be wise to request statistical assistance when utilizing these techniques.

Table 11.5   Tests That Control for the Impact of More than One Independent Variable on a Single Dependent Variable

Dependent Variable	Test	Example
Yes/No	Logistic Regression	Among adolescents who attempt to commit suicide, what is the relationship between alcohol consumption, age, gender, and risk of death? (Independent variables are alcohol consumption, age, and gender. Dependent variable is death (yes/no).
Continuous Variable	Multiple Regression	How do parents' education level, income level, and rank of school district affect fourth grade reading scores among impoverished children? (Independent variables are parents' education level, income level, and rank of school district. Dependent variable is reading score at the interval/ratio level.)

Interpreting Inferential Statistics

Obviously there are lots of different statistical tests available, and the one you use depends on what you are trying to determine. The good news is that, with the exception of the complexities involved in the regression techniques, each of these other tests produce a test statistic with a corresponding p value or probability value. The p value tells you the chance of observing what you are seeing in your sample if there is no relationship or association between the independent and dependent variables. If your study on New York State nurses determines the relationship between shift worked and job satisfaction has a p value of 0.02, then that means there is a 98% chance that there is an association between the shift worked and job satisfaction. There is only a 2% chance that the observations you collected occurred simply by chance.

The smaller the p value, the less the chance that your observations are just a chance occurrence and the greater the chance that there is an association or difference in the variables you are studying. When the p value of your test is less than the alpha you selected at the beginning of your study (usually 0.05), you are more certain there is a relationship than you said you needed to be at the beginning of your study. Consequently, you conclude there is a significant relationship between the variables you are studying. Stated more simply, a p value less than alpha means you have found a statistically significant relationship with any of these tests.

Understanding Clinical Significance

Notice that this testing determines *statistical* significance only. It doesn't say anything about *clinical* significance (also sometimes called *practical significance*). Clinical significance is a term that is frequently misused. In order to establish *clinical significance*, you must establish statistical significance, and then the experts in the field must weigh in on the topic to determine that the difference that is detected is important in a clinical setting.

For example, you might conduct a study that determines that individuals who ambulate post surgery utilizing the more expensive brand A walkers are significantly more likely to report high patient satisfaction scores but are discharged in the same time frame as those who use the less expensive brand B walkers. A statistically significant relationship is found between the type of walker utilized and the patient satisfaction level. However, when the clinical orthopedic experts read this information, they may feel that the difference is not clinically relevant because it did not affect the discharge time for the patients and the improvement in patient satisfaction was minimal. This is an example of a result that is statistically significant but not clinically significant. However, if there was a larger statistically significant improvement in patient satisfaction and also a statistically significant improvement in discharge times, the difference in discharge times could be clinically significant if the orthopedic experts believe they should change what the hospital is doing and order new brand A walkers. Statistical significance is determined using statistical analysis, whereas clinical significance is determined by experts in the field after statistical significance has been determined.

Q: *I've heard people say, "Well the results were not statistically significant, but they were clinically significant." What does that mean?*

A: There is no such thing! In order for there to be a clinically significant difference, there must be a statistically significant difference, which is then subjectively determined to be clinically relevant by the experts in the field.

Writing Your Research Proposal

After you have determined how you will analyze your research, you're ready to write it up in your proposal. Begin by stating the statistical program you will use, the sample you will collect, and the variables you will measure. Include demographic data and any population level data you have; also state how you will establish the representativeness of your sample. Note any distinct differences you anticipate finding in your sample compared to the general population data and the limits this could potentially create. Include your hypothesis and the variables you will evaluate to test it. Include the anticipated difference or effect size you hope to find using the literature you have read to support your estimation. Include how you have determined your sample size and why that is an adequate size for this study. Discuss the inferential statistics you will examine and any limitations that are anticipated in the collection of the data to support these methods. Include how your analysis is either unique or will address previously identified weaknesses in the literature. Be clear and concise. Analytical writing is not meant to be wordy or excessive. Say what you plan to do and then conclude.

Try It Now!

An infectious disease nurse directs a study to evaluate whether using pretreated antimicrobial Foley catheters decreases urinary bacterial counts upon removal compared to the standard untreated Foley catheters. She has a large surgical division with two side-by-side units (1500 East and 1500 West), which are staffed by the same group of nurses and receive the same base of patients. All incoming patients on 1500 East who need a Foley catheter receive the pretreated Foley catheters. The patients on 1500 West continue to have the standard Foley catheters as needed during the study. Urinary bacterial counts are determined upon removal of each Foley catheter.

After consulting with one of the hospital nurse researchers, the nurse decides to use an alpha of 0.05 and a power of 0.80. She needs to collect a sample of at least 1,200 patients. The study runs for 6 months, and at the end of the study the nurse notes that 670 patients with pretreated antimicrobial Foley catheters were cared for on 1500 East, and 712 patients with standard Foley catheters were cared for on 1500 West. A student t-test was used to compare the bacterial counts on the two units. The average urinary bacterial count on 1500 East was lower than on 1500 West with a *p* value of 0.02.

Question #1: Was the result statistically significant? Why or why not?

Yes, it was statistically significant because the *p* value was 0.02, which is less than the selected alpha of 0.05. This means there is only a 2% chance that these differences occurred by chance and the researcher was willing to accept up to a 5% chance (alpha of 0.05) that they occurred by chance. Thus, she concludes that there is a statistically significant difference in the bacterial counts on the two units.

Question #2: After completing further analysis the nurse determines that there is a statistically significant relationship between both the type of Foley catheter and the duration of time it is in place with the risk for an increased urinary bacterial count. She takes this information to the department chair, the hospital epidemiologist, the chief nursing officer, and the hospital CEO, who begin to take action to implement the recommendations of her study. She also publishes the study in *Clinical Infectious Diseases*. Why is her work now considered clinically significant?

First, the study has established statistical significance. Further, each of these individuals, who are experts in their field, believes action should be taken regarding these findings, which is sufficient to establish clinical significance. The publication by a reputable professional journal also supports the argument for clinical significance.

References

Edwards, A. (n.d.). Some quotations by R. A. Fisher. Retrieved from http://www.economics.soton.ac.uk/staff/aldrich/fisherguide/quotations.htm

Heavey, E. (2013). *Statistics for nursing: A practical approach* (2nd ed.). Sudbury, MA: Jones and Bartlett Publishing.

Munro, B. (2005). *Statistical methods for health care research* (5th ed.). New York: Lippincott Williams & Wilkins.

Polit, D. (2010). *Statistics and data analysis for nursing research* (2nd ed.). Upper Saddle River, NJ: Pearson.

Tufte, E. (2001). *Visual display of quantitative information* (2nd ed., p.80). Cheshire, CT: Graphics Press.

"Words do two major things:
They provide food for the mind and create light
for understanding and awareness."

–Jim Rohn

Qualitative Research

Barbara Williams

12

Previous chapters have described the quantitative method of research—how to use numbers in order to quantify your data. This chapter discusses qualitative research—how to use words to learn more about a particular concept, or *phenomenon*. The data in qualitative research is composed largely of words rather than numbers. To better understand this difference, let's look at a clinical situation.

You are caring for a patient, Mrs. Fisher, who has rheumatoid arthritis and has a considerable amount of pain. In order to medicate her for pain, you ask her to rate it on a scale from zero to ten, with ten being the worst pain possible. She tells you it is an "eight," and so you medicate her accordingly. You have used a number to objectively quantify her pain. Suppose, however, you want to know *how* Mrs. Fisher experiences her pain, so you ask her, "What is it like to suffer the pain of rheumatoid arthritis?" She may tell you that it is very difficult to move because of the pain, and the simple task of getting dressed takes a considerable amount of time. She may further explain that she doesn't like to take a lot of pain medication because of the side effects and that gardening was her favorite hobby, but she is no longer able to enjoy it because it is too painful. In addition, the pain prevents her from cooking, and so her husband has had to take over that household task. He is not a good cook, and this causes frustration for both of them.

WHAT YOU'LL LEARN IN THIS CHAPTER

- Whereas quantitative research uses numbers to determine relationships among concepts, qualitative research uses words to learn more about a concept, or phenomenon.

- Qualitative research is important because it allows us to understand an event, circumstance, or situation from the perspective of those who have experienced it.

- The qualitative research process has some similarities to quantitative research, including devising a research question, recruiting a sample, and collecting and analyzing data.

Rather than using an instrument to measure "how much" pain Mrs. Fisher has, you have asked a question to learn more about what it means for her to "experience" pain as she lives her everyday life. You have expanded your understanding of pain for this patient. This is an essential difference between quantitative and qualitative research: *quantitative* uses numbers to answer a question whereas *qualitative* uses words. This chapter explains more about the difference between quantitative and qualitative methods and about the uses of qualitative research in clinical practice. It also describes specific qualitative designs and how to evaluate qualitative evidence.

What Is Qualitative Research?

If you take the preceding example about the fictitious Mrs. Fisher and transpose it from a clinical situation to a research study, it becomes apparent that qualitative research seeks to elicit the experiences of the participants, through their own words, so that you can understand the meaning that the situation or event has for them. Rich descriptions from participants, in as much detail as possible, and observations by the researcher provide much of the data in a qualitative study.

Another major difference between qualitative and quantitative research is in regard to the stance of the researcher. In quantitative research, the researcher defines the concept(s) to be measured (independent variable) and identifies the outcome he/she will be looking for (dependent variable; see Chapter 4). In qualitative research the approach is one of openness. The researcher is seeking a broader description of the phenomenon and does not hypothesize about an outcome. The outcome emerges as the study progresses. In qualitative research the participant is the expert, and it is the job of the researcher to listen and to learn.

Why Do Qualitative Research?

Qualitative research is useful for guiding nursing practice, building nursing theory, and contributing to instrument development (Barroso, 2010). Findings can be useful to nurses in the clinical setting. One example is a study conducted by Karlsson, Bergbom, and Forsberg (2011), who inquired about patients' experiences of being conscious while mechanically ventilated. They interviewed 12 participants after they were discharged from the intensive care unit (ICU). The findings indicated that participants endured a sense of panic at being "breathless," at being unable to talk, and at being completely dependent on technology and caregivers for survival. They felt helpless, deserted, and powerless. It was important for them to be able to communicate with nurses and family and to regain their independence. Participating in their care decreased their sense of dependency and made them feel part of the team. Talking about life outside the ICU increased their hope for survival.

This was an important study because nurses in the ICU who care for this patient population can gain greater insight to what patients experience and tailor their care to those strategies that facilitate communication, emotional comfort, independence, and recovery. Results from this study, then, can influence nursing practice. Furthermore, there would be no other way to obtain this information except to ask those who have experienced it.

Another example comes from a study about the experience of hope in patients who had an acute spinal cord injury (Lohne & Severinsson, 2005). The researchers interviewed 10 participants in a rehabilitation facility in the first few months after the injury in order to understand what "hope" meant to them. Hope was defined as "future oriented toward improvements" (p. 285). All participants expressed hope in terms of longing for their lives as they were before the accident. A deeper view of hope revealed a movement between such inner emotional dichotomies as inner strength and vulnerability; pride and shame; despair and happiness; courage and uncertainty; and patience and restlessness. Hope seemed to give energy and direction for the future. Based on the findings, the researchers concluded that nurses need the skills to foster hope and enable recently injured patients to look beyond the immediate situation and direct their energies appropriately to the future.

It is also important to understand the perspective of nurses and other health care professionals through qualitative research designs. Eggenberger (2012) conducted a qualitative study on the role of the charge nurse in the acute care setting. She interviewed 20 charge nurses or assistant nurse managers at 4 hospitals about the experience of their roles. The themes that emerged from the interviews suggested that the charge nurse role had an effect on patient safety; the timeliness, efficiency, and effectiveness of care; and patient satisfaction. As the researcher concluded, nurse executives can use the findings to stress the importance of this role to the organization. Often these support roles are not considered cost effective and are frequently analyzed to determine if they are essential to care.

The importance of qualitative research to instrument development is evident in the work of Beck, a nurse scientist. She interviewed 7 women about their experiences of postpartum depression (PPD) (Beck, 1992). The women described 11 themes that captured their experience, including unbearable loneliness, contemplating death, obsessive thoughts, fear and guilt about pondering harming their babies, uncontrollable anxiety, and feeling like a robot.

Beck pointed out that prior to her study, previous research on PPD used a quantitative design with instruments comprised of items that may have been descriptive of depression in general, but were not congruent with the descriptions of PPD from women who had the experience. She concluded that the findings from her qualitative study could be a starting point for the development of a quantitative instrument to specifically measure PPD. After Beck (1993) conducted another qualitative study on postpartum depression, Beck and Gable (2000, 2001a, 2001b) developed and assessed the validity of the Postpartum Depression Screening Scale using items created from Beck's qualitative studies.

The Qualitative Research Process

This section describes the qualitative research process. This is meant as an introduction to the method so that you can have some familiarity with it. Obviously, not everything about a research method can be contained in one short chapter. Furthermore, if you have no experience in conducting qualitative research (or any research), you should not attempt to conduct a study on your own. But if you have a topic in mind that you would like to investigate, there are some things you can do.

You first need to know if your department/organization will support the study. You might want to check with your colleagues, your manager, and/or your department head to see if they are interested in knowing more about the topic. Then you will need to investigate the resources that are available to you:

- Are there opportunities to learn more about the qualitative research process?

- Is there someone with experience in qualitative research in your organization who can mentor you?

- If not, is there a researcher at a nearby university or in your professional organization who may help?

You should make sure that you have the necessary education and sufficient guidance before you begin a study. In our organization's clinical advancement program (clinical ladder) for staff nurses, a segment of the top tier of the program is comprised of Specialty Scholars. They are staff nurses who agree to conduct either quality improvement, research, or evidence-based practice (EBP) projects. They attend a three-day core curriculum in order to learn the skills needed to lead such projects and then are assigned a mentor to guide them through the completion of the project.

For example, three staff nurses, who were research scholars, wanted to conduct a qualitative study about the experience of health care professionals in the emergency department when that department moved to a new location. Prior to writing their proposal, they attended the core curriculum, learned about the research process, and then were guided on the development of the proposal and through every step of the study by a nurse scientist who had previous experience conducting qualitative research.

The Research Question

The choice about whether or not to conduct a qualitative study depends on what you want to know and the question you are seeking to answer. Qualitative inquiry seeks to understand experiences, behaviors, and processes. Questions may begin with:

- "What is the essence of...?"

- "What is the nature of...?"

- What is the lived experience of...?"

- "What is the process of...?"

For instance, using our earlier example, if you were to conduct a qualitative study about pain in women with rheumatoid arthritis, then your question might be, "What is the lived experience of pain in women suffering from rheumatoid arthritis?" As you see later in this chapter, the phrasing of the question will depend on the type of qualitative study you choose to do.

Q: *Is the process of developing a research question for a qualitative study the same as for a quantitative study?*

A: In qualitative research the research question does not contain independent and dependent variables as a quantitative research question would. The question in qualitative research is open and broad as the researcher learns the answer, or outcome, from the participants in the study.

Qualitative Sampling

In qualitative research the gold standard is not random sampling as it is quantitative research. In qualitative research you want to recruit participants who can provide information in detail about the phenomenon (or particular concept) of interest. If possible, you will also want to vary that sample as much as possible in regard to characteristics such as gender, age, and ethnicity. This is not for the purpose of generalizing your results, but to get the most comprehensive description of the phenomena.

In qualitative research the idea is not to obtain as large a sample as possible or to predetermine the sample size by techniques such as power analysis. Samples sizes tend to be small and are determined by what's called *data saturation* (Mauk, 2012a; Polit & Beck, 2010). Data saturation is the point at which you are hearing no new information. Remember that the goal is to describe the phenomenon in as much detail as possible so that you can have as broadened an understanding as possible. You are interested in depth, not breadth. Although sample sizes are small, you might need to interview participants more than once to attain depth of information (read more about depth of information later in this chapter). Interview times may vary, but it is not unusual for them to last an hour or more. And, believe it or not, the interviews can generate a considerable amount of data.

Q: *How does a qualitative researcher manage such a large amount of data?*

A: There are methods for managing and reducing large amounts of data by breaking them into smaller segments and moving from particular descriptions to general statements. This process starts soon after data collection is begun, before too much data accumulates. You will learn more about how this is accomplished later in this chapter.

Data Collection

Interviews and observation are the main sources of data collection in qualitative research. An interview guide is often used, but the purpose is not to control the interview; the guide is designed to provide items for discussion. As the goal is obtaining as rich a description as possible, it is important to ask questions in a way that you can obtain as much information as possible. That means refraining from questions that can be answered by "yes" or "no" or by one-word answers. Asking open-ended questions is the best way to obtain the most information. These are questions that answer who, what, when, where, why, and how. For example rather than asking a question such as, "Was your pain addressed adequately?" you might ask, "What, if anything, was done to manage your pain?" or "How was your pain managed?" You can also ask follow-up questions such as, "What was that like for you?" or, "How did you feel about that?" to obtain more information.

There is one important step that qualitative researchers must take that quantitative researchers do not have to be as concerned with. As you collect and analyze your data, it is important in qualitative research to be able to separate what you already know or think about the phenomenon from what the participants are telling you about the phenomenon. For example, imagine you decide to conduct a study on the experience of pain in patients who have rheumatoid arthritis. You have read the literature about pain in this population, and you have had clinical experience with such patients. After all, Mrs. Fisher, your patient, has told you what it is like. One of the things she told you is that her husband has to do the cooking and that is frustrating for both of them.

You are now interviewing a woman in your study about her experience with pain in rheumatoid arthritis, and she tells you that her husband has to do all the cooking. When she tells you this you think to yourself, "Mmm…that has to be frustrating for her." You have made an assumption based on your previous experience. In order to avoid making assumptions, it is important that you be aware of your own knowledge, opinions, and experiences so that they don't interfere with your ability to truly hear and understand the experience of the participants. Otherwise, you will run the risk of producing results that are merely reflections of your own thinking. Many qualitative researchers write down their previous knowledge and opinions prior to data collection.

Q: *When I am reading a qualitative study, how do I know if the researcher has acknowledged his/her preconceived knowledge, experience, and opinions?*

A: Sometimes the researcher states in the article that he/she has done so and describes their preconceptions. However, more often, given the word count allowed in most journals, that information is not included. The researcher must make choices about what information is the most important to convey in the space allotted. That being said, you can look for other information in the article to determine if researcher bias has unduly influenced the findings. For example, how did the researcher establish trustworthiness? Did he/she have another researcher independently analyze the data and arrive at similar conclusions? Did he/she return to the participants to have them validate the findings? Are there sufficient verbatim quotes from participants that are congruent with the findings established by the researcher?

So now let's say you have made notes of your preconceived knowledge. Your thoughts as you are interviewing your study participant may go something like this: "Gee. Mrs. Fisher said that her husband does the cooking, and it is frustrating. I should ask further questions about what this is like for this person." So you ask your participant, "What is it like for you to have your husband do all the cooking?" She may respond, "I love it. He is a great cook." In this example, your previous knowledge has guided your question, but you have refrained from assuming the answer.

Taping Your Interviews

When collecting data in interviews, it is best to audiotape them. Your data will be more accurate, and you will be able to focus on what participants are saying rather than be distracted by trying to write everything down or remember it later. In order to avoid the participant being intimidated by this, it is important to tell them that anything that they say during the interview, but don't want included in the study, will be erased.

During qualitative interviewing, the researcher engages in observations about such factors as the setting; interactions that occur during the interview; and the participants' appearance, nonverbal behavior, and response to the researcher (Hoskins & Mariano, 2004a). Immediately, or as soon as possible after the interview, the researcher is encouraged to write down these observations in what are called *field notes*. These observations become part of the data and help to place the participant's words within a broader context. This information can be very important in uncovering meaning that is embedded in the data.

Other Methods of Data Collection

Although interviews and observation are the main methods of data collection, other methods, including artwork, photographs, diaries, and documents, may be used that can then lead to a deeper understanding of what an experience means to a participant (Hoskins & Mariano, 2004a).

It may be necessary, in qualitative research, to conduct more than one interview with each participant. This is done to obtain more information and to clarify and verify the information already obtained. Many times a participant will remember something important that he/she didn't mention in the first interview. Additional interviews give the participants the opportunity to include this information. If you are a nurse working in the acute care setting and want to conduct a qualitative study in that setting, it is important to remember that the patient may be discharged by the time you want to conduct the second interview, so the second interview might have to take place in another setting (outpatient department, home, sub-acute, etc.) or by telephone.

In addition to individual interviews, qualitative research can be conducted in focus groups. Focus group interviews involve groups of 5 to 10 participants who are brought together to explore thoughts about a particular topic. A moderator, who uses an interview guide, guides participants in the discussion. Through group interaction, insights can develop that might not arise in individual interviews (Dougherty, 2012). However, one drawback is that many people do not feel comfortable expressing their thoughts in front of a group (Polit & Beck, 2010).

Data Analysis

Many methods exist for data analysis in qualitative research, but generally speaking analysis is a process of identifying patterns, commonalities, and regularities in the transcribed interviews. Unlike quantitative research, data collection and analysis occur simultaneously in qualitative research. The following describes one method: After one interview is transcribed, you begin analysis. You first read the entire transcript and then listen to the recorded interview while reading the transcribed version. This is very important—you may notice voice tones and voice inflections that escaped notice during the interview. Also, some parts of participants' responses that did not seem important at the time might take on greater importance when you listen to them in the context of the whole interview. This also gives you an opportunity to correct any mistakes in the transcription.

After you have reviewed the transcripts, you attempt to make meaning of the data by breaking it down into smaller segments. Note words, phrases, or sentences that stand out and assign a code to them; then cluster similar codes into categories (Mariano 1995; Hoskins & Mariano, 2004b). For example, in a study about the experiences of patients who received stem cell transplants (Williams, 2008), descriptions from several participants such as, "I just felt strange in my body;" "Somebody else…took over my body;" and, "It's almost like an out-of-body experience" could all be assigned the code "identity." These descriptions could then be clustered into the category "Participants perceived an altered relationship to their bodies." This movement from specific details to a general statement is the process of *data reduction*. The researcher must make decisions about what pieces of data are most representative of the whole story (Mauk, 2012b).

Repeat this process for each piece of data. After you have analyzed three or four interviews, you cluster common categories together to formulate themes. You analyze subsequent interviews using the themes you've developed. If the data does not reflect the initial themes, then you change the themes to better reflect the data. Continue until all the interviews are analyzed and a comprehensive description of the phenomenon emerges (Mariano 1995; Hoskins & Mariano, 2004b). This process is akin to putting pieces of a puzzle together, and it should form a meaningful picture of the participants' stories (Mauk, 2012b).

Types of Qualitative Research

So far we have been looking at a general description of qualitative research. This section briefly covers some of the different types of qualitative research, known as the *research traditions*. Three traditions, derived from different disciplines, are prominent in qualitative nursing research (Polit & Beck, 2010):

- Phenomenology, which derives from philosophy

- Grounded theory, which derives from sociology

- Ethnography, which derives from anthropology

These traditions are frameworks; that is, they "frame" the study process. Each asks a different question, has a different focus, and employs a different method. There are also somewhat different methods for collecting and analyzing data *within* each tradition. The important thing to remember is that the method must be consistent with the framework and that you follow the chosen method.

Phenomenology

Phenomenology is rooted in phenomenological philosophy. The researcher's goal is to understand the "lived experience" from the perception of those living it. It asks the question, "What is the essence of the experience?" or "What is the lived experience (of the phenomenon)?" The studies cited earlier by Karlsson et al. (2011), Lohne & Severinsson (2005), and Beck (1992) are examples of phenomenological studies because they sought to understand what it was like for participants to live through a particular experience.

Grounded Theory

Grounded theory derives from sociology and focuses on processes within a social setting. It asks, "What is the process of this phenomenon?" From the data, the researcher develops codes and categories to build a theory (that's why it is called *grounded*) that explains the phenomenon. In this type of study, the researcher seeks to identify the main process and the behaviors that are used to resolve it (Polit & Beck, 2010).

An example is a study conducted by Runquist (2006) about postpartum fatigue. She interviewed 13 women between 2 and 5 weeks postpartum. She identified "persevering" as the central process of postpartum fatigue. Participants persevered in caregiving of infants and older children in spite of an overwhelming desire to rest. They used coping behaviors and the belief that children brought purpose and meaning to their lives to resolve the problem. The theory was titled "Persevering through Postpartum Fatigue" and contributed to a deeper understanding of the phenomenon of postpartum fatigue.

Q: *I am interested in studying the process that nurses in our hospital use in their unit-based councils to resolve unit problems. What type of study should I do?*

A: This topic would best be addressed by using a qualitative study design. More specifically, it calls for grounded theory methodology. Grounded theory is used when one wants to study a social process and patterns of interaction that are used to solve problems. It results in an actual theory that is grounded in the data provided by the study participants.

Ethnography

Ethnography derives from anthropology and focuses on cultural patterns and experiences. The purpose is to understand the shared meanings that shape the behavior of a group. It asks the question, "What is the culture of this group of people?" The researcher comes to understand the culture of others by entering the world of the study participants "to watch what happens, listen to what is said, and collect whatever data is available" (Barroso, 2010, p. 109).

In ethnography, the researcher spends a considerable amount of time observing behaviors in the culture and talking informally to members of the culture in addition to conducting interviews. This is known as *participant observation.* As an outsider the researcher seeks to understand the worldview of the participants (emic view) and contrasts it with the researcher's view (etic view). A culture can be a certain ethnic group, a group of nurses who work on a particular unit, or a group of patients who share a particular diagnosis.

For example, Lauzon Clabo (2008) conducted an ethnographic study on the assessment of pain across two surgical units. Data were collected through observation, individual interviews, and focus group discussions with nurses on each unit. Nurses on Unit One were consistent in their approach, which was to rely predominantly on objective data such as the type of surgery and the amount of pain expected with that surgery. Nurses on Unit Two were also consistent in their approach. However, they relied predominantly on subjective data—the patient's report of pain. From the observations and interviews, the researcher concluded that each unit had a distinctly different pattern of pain assessment that was shaped by the culture, or the social context, of that unit.

Ethical Standards

Ethical standards that apply to quantitative studies also apply to qualitative studies. However, because of the nature of qualitative inquiry, there are some additional precautions that you must consider. Here are the main considerations. Depending on the interview material, participants may become emotional during an interview. If that occurs you should:

- Ask the participant if he/she would like you to turn off the tape recorder or erase anything that has been recorded.

- Ask the participant if he/she wants to stop the interview.

- Consider a referral to a counselor if the participant is particularly upset.

When audiotapes are transcribed, you must replace any identifying information (such as name, address, place of employment, or phone numbers) with fictitious information (Mauk, 2012a). However, that is not enough. Even though fictitious information is used, qualitative research studies include "rich description" which in and of itself can reveal identity. You must take extra precaution to safeguard identity when reporting the results of the study (Polit & Beck, 2010). For example, if a participant in a study happens to be a public official, such as the town mayor, you would not reveal details of his/her employment or details about the town in your findings that could reveal his/her identity even if this material is revealed by the participant in the recorded data.

Evaluating Qualitative Research

Criteria such as internal and external validity, generalizability, reliability, and objectivity are not used in qualitative methods. Nevertheless, qualitative studies need to be conducted with a high degree of rigor because of the potential for bias that is inherent in this type of study. Qualitative researchers are required to establish trustworthiness, which is the degree to which the reader can have confidence in the results of the study (Mauk, 2012b). The following are some of the ways that you can establish trustworthiness based on the criteria established by Lincoln and Guba (1985):

- Have another researcher as well as investigator analyze the data and then compare the themes identified. Discuss and adjust the themes until a common understanding of the data is reached. This is called *peer debriefing*.

- Send the data, themes, and the method used to develop themes to a researcher knowledgeable about qualitative research (auditor) who can then follow "the trail" to determine if the process used to develop the themes is logical. This is known as an *audit trail*.

- Use ample verbatim participant quotes to support the themes.

- Return to the participants to ask them if the themes generated from the interviews are consistent with their experience. Any changes suggested by the participants should be incorporated in the findings. This is called *member checking*.

- Discern if the results of the study can be applied to another context or situation. This is known as *transferability*.

When you evaluate a study that is rooted in one of the research traditions we discussed earlier, it is important to consider if the researcher followed the method that is consistent with the tradition. For example, in an ethnographic study, did the researcher engage in participant observation of behavior as well as conduct interviews? In a grounded theory study, did the researcher describe a social process rather than a lived experience?

You should keep in mind that within the qualitative research paradigm there are many methods and many variations in data collection techniques and data analysis. This chapter is intended to give you a basic understanding of qualitative research in general and some of the methods within it. Hopefully this will spark your interest in reading a qualitative study or perhaps conducting a qualitative study yourself with the appropriate guidance.

Try It Now!

Mary is a staff nurse on an oncology unit. She had noticed a while ago that when patients are admitted to the unit they are very anxious. She has been offering them relaxation tapes that are comprised of music and relaxation exercises. Anecdotally, Mary has observed that these have been very helpful to the patients who have used them. Now she would like to conduct a qualitative study in order to find out what the patients' experiences are when they use the tapes. Before approaching a researcher from the nursing research committee for assistance, Mary starts to think about how she would go about this. She decides that her research question will be, "What is the effectiveness of relaxation tapes on anxiety in patients admitted to an oncology unit?"

Next, Mary thinks about how she will interview the participants, so she writes down some questions:

1. Did the tapes relax you?

2. How long did the relaxation last?

3. How many times did you use them?

4. Would you use the tapes again the next time you come to the hospital?

Mary thinks that she can do this study pretty quickly. She knows that in qualitative studies, the sample sizes are small, so she decides that she will only need to interview 5 participants. Excited about proceeding with the study now that she has some ideas, Mary sets up an appointment with the nurse researcher. You are the researcher Mary contacts. What would you tell her about her thoughts so far?

First you would congratulate Mary on her observations and on her desire to do research. Then you would help Mary understand the following:

- The question is not appropriate for a qualitative study. It has an independent variable (relaxation tapes) and dependent variable (anxiety) and suggests she will test the effectiveness of one on the other. If this is what Mary wants to do she should do a quantitative study and use a tool to measure anxiety. But if she wants to know how the participants experience the relaxation tapes then she should do a qualitative study and her question would be, "What is the experience of using relaxation tapes in patients on an oncology unit?"

- The questions may not yield very rich descriptions as they can be answered by "yes" or "no" or one-word answers. You can help Mary devise questions that can elicit more data such as:

  - "What was it like to listen to the relaxation tapes?"

  - "How did you feel after you listened to them?"

  - "What, if anything, would you change about the tape if you could?"

- In qualitative studies, sample size is not determined prior to data collection and analysis. It is determined by data saturation: There is no new information forthcoming.

References

Barroso, J. (2010). Qualitative approaches to research. In G. LoBiondo-Wood & J. Haber (Eds.), *Nursing research* (7th ed.). (pp. 100–125). St. Louis, MO: Mosby.

Beck, C. (1992). The lived experience of postpartum depression: A phenomenological study. *Nursing Research, 41*(3), 166–170.

Beck, C. (1993). Teetering on the edge: A substantive theory of postpartum depression. *Nursing Research, 42*(1), 42–48.

Beck, C., & Gable, R. (2000). Postpartum depression screening scale: Development and psychometric testing. *Nursing Research, 49*(5), 272–282.

Beck, C., & Gable, R. (2001a). Further validation of the postpartum depression screening scale. *Nursing Research, 50*(3), 155-164.

Beck, C., & Gable, R. (2001b). Comparative analysis of the performance of the postpartum depression screening scale with two other depression instruments. *Nursing Research, 50*(4), 242–250.

Dougherty, J. (2012). Data collection: Planning and piloting. In N. Schmidt & J. M. Brown (Eds.), *Evidence-based practice for nurses* (2nd ed.). (pp. 217–245). Sudbury, MA: Jones & Bartlett.

Eggenberger, T. (2012). Exploring the charge nurse role: Holding the frontline. *The Journal of Nursing Administration, 42*(11), 502–506. doi: 0.1097/NNA.0b013e3182714495

Hoskins, C. N., & Mariano, C. (2004a). Research designs. In C. N. Hoskins & C. Mariano (Eds.), *Research in nursing and health* (2nd ed.). (pp. 28–39). New York: Springer.

Hoskins, C. N., & Mariano, C. (2004b). Data analysis and interpretation. In C.N. Hoskins & C. Mariano (Eds.), *Research in nursing and health* (2nd ed.). (pp. 60–68). New York: Springer.

Karlsson, V., Bergbom, I., & Forsberg, A. (2011). The lived experience of adult intensive care patients who were conscious during mechanical ventilation: A phenomenological-hermeneutic study. *Intensive and Critical Care Nursing, 28*(1), 6–15. doi: 10.1016/j.1ccn.2011.11.002

Lauzon Clabo, L. M. (2008). An ethnography of pain assessment and the role of social context on two postoperative units. *Journal of Advanced Nursing, 61*(5), 531–539.

Lincoln, Y. S., & Guba, E. G. (1985). *Naturalistic inquiry.* Newbury Park, CA: Sage.

Lohne, V., & Severinsson, E. (2005). Hope during the first months after acute spinal cord injury. *Issues and Innovations in Nursing Practice, 47*(3), 279–286.

Mariano, C. (1995). The qualitative research process. In L. Talbot (Ed.), *Principles and practices of nursing research,* (pp. 463–489). St. Louis, MO: Mosby.

Mauk, K. (2012a). Qualitative designs: Using words to provide evidence. In N. Schmidt & J. M. Brown (Eds.), *Evidence-based practice for nurses* (2nd ed.). (pp. 187–215). Sudbury, MA: Jones & Bartlett.

Mauk, K. (2012b). What do the qualitative data mean? In N. Schmidt & J. M. Brown (Eds.) *Evidence-based practice for nurses* (2nd ed.). (pp. 341–375). Sudbury, MA: Jones & Bartlett.

Polit, D. F., & Beck, C. T. (2010). *Essentials of nursing research: Appraising evidence for nursing practice* (7th ed.). Philadelphia, PA: Wolters Kluwer Health Lippincott Williams & Wilkins.

Rohn, J. (n.d.). BrainyQuote.com. Retrieved http://www.brainyquote.com/quotes/quotes/j/jimrohn121687.html

Runquist, J. (2006). Persevering through postpartum fatigue. *JOGNN, 36*(1), 28–37. doi: 10.1111/J.1552-6909.2006.00116.x

Williams, B. (2008). *Rebirth: The experience of self-transcendence in patients who have undergone stem cell transplantation.* (Doctoral dissertation). New York University, New York.

*"No study is complete
until the findings have been shared."*

–Denise Polit and Cheryl Beck

Dissemination: The Last Frontier

Margo A. Halm

13

You may consider presenting your findings at local, regional, or national professional conferences, or you may desire to write your findings for publication in a research, general, or specialty-based practice journal. But you might be wondering, "Why is spreading the results of my research so important?" There are many answers to this question. Dissemination is the last phase of the research process. It enables you to share newly generated knowledge and contribute to the larger body of knowledge. This collective body of knowledge on your topic builds the discipline of nursing and demonstrates the effect of your profession on patient outcomes. This chapter discusses what you need to know about the final phase of the research process, known as *dissemination*. Dissemination starts with the creation of an abstract to provide a succinct overview of your research study. Once developed, you'll use your abstract to request presenting your research findings at conferences, in either poster or podium sessions, as well as in any publications you write for professional journals.

Presenting Research Results

Think of dissemination as similar to communicating the results of tests/procedures to patients. Doing so helps patients comprehend their health condition and treatments. With research, the need to

WHAT YOU'LL LEARN IN THIS CHAPTER

- Whether presenting your study as a poster or at a podium, it's important to take the time to develop a strong abstract.

- Poster presentations provide a dynamic opportunity to share the results of your research.

- Presentations at the podium provide a rich opportunity to share your research findings at general or specialty-based nursing conferences.

disseminate findings assists your colleagues—both within and outside nursing—to understand how the new knowledge can be used in clinical practice.

Beyond building the discipline, dissemination has professional benefits. First, dissemination provides you with rich opportunities to network and learn from colleagues with similar interests who often provide sage advice for further development of your research. Such sharing can lead to collaborative research opportunities. Completion of each phase of the research process builds different professional skills/abilities that contribute to your growth as a professional within your subspecialty. Thus, building dissemination skills assists you to find your voice and tell your research story!

How can you get started on the path toward dissemination? Begin thinking about your purpose and intended audience: Will it be a podium or poster presentation at a local/regional/national conference or a written research report in a professional journal? After you have made this decision, you need to write the research abstract. It is extremely important to follow all abstract instructions very carefully before you submit it.

Q: *If I submit an abstract for a conference, can I choose either a poster or podium presentation? If accepted, will my registration be waived?*

A: It depends. Some conferences are very prescriptive in their call for abstracts and ask authors to specify if their interest lies in either a podium or poster presentation. Some may also give authors a choice to say either podium or poster and the conference planners then decide the forum. Others may leave it open to their discretion, informing prospective authors of their right to choose presentation style. In relation to registration fees, many conferences (but not all) will offer a reduced fee to accepted presenters. Check the call-for-abstract information or call the conference sponsors to be sure.

All Roads Begin With an Abstract

What is a research abstract? A *research abstract* is a brief but complete written synopsis of your research project. Writing an abstract involves succinctly describing the problem, as well as key methods, results, and conclusions of your project. Think of the abstract as similar to a surgical report that specifies the procedure performed, reason for the procedure, surgical techniques used, key findings, and how the patient tolerated the procedure. Research abstracts are the key material that conference organizers use to determine if a body of work is chosen for oral or poster presentation.

Q: *Who reviews abstracts submitted to conferences? Is this process blind?*

A: Conference sponsors generally have a panel or committee of member volunteers who review and score submitted abstracts. A list of criteria or a scoring grid is typically used to make the review process as objective as possible. The abstract review process is most commonly blinded, which means that all personally identifiable author information has been removed from the abstract submission before the abstracts are released to the review panel.

Where should you present your research? Wood and Morrison (2011) advocated that authors contemplate what audience will be most interested in the topic, as well as which conference will provide the best opportunity for networking and potential future collaboration. Another question to ask is whether a particular theme of a conference is a good fit with your research. Your research mentor is also an excellent source of information about conference options, so don't hesitate to seek that person's advice.

After you narrow your options, review abstracts that were accepted at last year's conference (Wood & Morrison, 2011). Most conferences publish abstracts in proceeding books or the professional journals of the sponsoring association. Knowing the venue where you will present enables you to plan for your prospective audience, such as the likely size and whether formal or informal language is used (Norwood, 2000). Think about how you can tailor the abstract depending on whether your audience is comprised of only nurses, or it includes professionals from other clinical disciplines and roles (i.e., educators, researchers, administrators). If the audience is clinicians, emphasize clinical implications and not recommendations for further research (which researchers in the field would be keen to learn). Clearly, each group will look at your research from a different angle, enlarging your learning in different ways. As Polit and Beck (2012) pointed out, researchers often need to write for multiple audiences and, thus, need a multipronged strategy.

Next, scrutinize the call-for-abstracts/journal guidelines as these documents provide specific instructions on how to prepare the abstract. Regardless of the venue—conference or journal—following the guidelines cannot be overemphasized. The guidelines specify the type of abstract required (structured or unstructured), rules related to titles, word/character limit, formatting (fonts, margins/spacing, tables/figures), and submission deadlines. If possible, track down the abstract review criteria used by conference sponsors. Research abstracts are generally critiqued on the basis of content; quality; contributions to nursing scholarship, theory and/or practice; originality; and clarity/completeness (Norwood, 2000).

Abstract submission for conferences is usually online. Check the instructions to discover whether the abstract should be submitted as an attachment to a specified email address or on a web-based system with preset fields and word limits. Conference organizers will inquire about your preference (poster, podium, or either). The status of your research is another consideration with conferences. Whereas completed research may be accepted for either poster or podium presentation, typically research that remains in process is granted poster presentation only. Furthermore, most conferences do not allow research that has been previously published to be presented (Wood & Morrison, 2011).

Abstract Content

A common anatomical structure used for research abstracts is what is referred to as the IMRAD (Introduction, Methods, Results, and Discussion) method (Norwood, 2000; Polit & Beck, 2012):

- **Introduction:** The "Introduction" specifies why the project was done. Provide a concise description of the problem and its significance to nursing, followed by the study purpose and research questions/hypotheses.

- **Methods:** The "Methods" section describes what was done (design, sample/setting, instruments, intervention).

- **Results:** The "Results" section captures key findings mapped to each research question.

- **Discussion:** The "Discussion" section explains key conclusions and implications for practice/further research.

Q: *Do I need to include my references in my abstract?*

A: No. References are not included in abstracts.

The Title

Choose an eye-catching title to not only capture interest but also to communicate the clinical importance of your research. Think of the title as a tool to sell the study's importance just as the title of a patient education brochure entices your patient to want to learn. Short, informative titles that include an action verb are most engaging (no more than 10 to 12 words) (Briggs, 2009; Ellerbee, 2006; Miller, 2007; Wood & Morrison, 2011). Make sure to list most important terms first, and avoid acronyms or any unnecessary phrases such as "a study of" or "an investigation into" in the title.

Structure

Abstracts are structured or unstructured. "Structured" abstracts require subheadings for sections (see Figure 13.1). Such headings are some variation of the IMRAD method, so use those provided in the conference/journal guidelines. Although IMRAD is a great tool for learning the basic anatomy of a research abstract, every conference or journal has its own specific styles and structures. On the other hand, "unstructured" abstracts cover the same elements but contain no headings (see Figure 13.2).

Style Considerations

Other rules of thumb for abstracts include use of an active voice and the third person. Limit jargon and abbreviations (spell them out the first time you use them). Don't sweat the word limit at first. Write a first draft and then critically review the content to whittle it down to the most critical information. Plan to read/reread your abstract to achieve clarity and conciseness. It is always helpful to have an experienced colleague critique your abstract (Wood & Morrison, 2011). Abstract reviewers will look for authors who follow directions and write a clear abstract that is easy to understand, where all pieces are linked. As a result, findings and conclusions need to be based on your results, as well as be internally consistent with the methods.

 What style guidelines should researchers typically follow?

 It depends. Some call for abstracts and publications use the American Psychological Association (APA) guidelines, but others use the American Medication Association (AMA) citation style. Thus, this question reinforces the need for authors to follow the abstract or journal guidelines carefully as citation style instructions will be dictated.

Introduction: While frequent ED users account for a small percentage of ED visits, these patients can drain the system, contributing to overcrowding and lowered quality of care.

Methods: This retrospective descriptive correlational study explored characteristics of frequent ED users at a large Midwestern urban hospital, and factors predictive of high ED utilization. The sample included adult patients with at least 6 visits in 2005-2006 (N=201). For each, 6 visits were randomly chosen for chart review (N=1200 visits) of demographic, health history and clinical factors such as chief complaints.

Results: Frequent users were commonly female, 35 years old, Caucasian, single, unemployed, living alone, with private insurance/Medicaid, and a primary care physician. Top chief complaints were: Abdominal pain, headache, chest pain, low back pain, and lower extremity pain. However, a Poisson regression found male, non-Black race, part-time employment, retired/unemployed, Medicare, and chief complaint of upper respiratory infection were associated with a higher number of ED visits. Headache approached significance as an independent predictor of more visits.

Discussion: Almost 95% had <10 ED visits/year, with pain the overall top chief complaint. Seventy percent of frequent visits occurred on either the evening or night shift, perhaps indicating access issues to primary physician or urgent care clinics. The rate of frequent users was comparable to other investigations yet, few similarities in patient characteristics and predictors of high emergency department utilization were found, partly due to the retrospective design, but certainly reinforcing limited generalizability of ED utilization patterns across centers in different metropolitan and geographic regions (*Journal of Emergency Nursing*, 2009).

Reprinted with permission.

Figure 13.1   Exemplar for a structured research abstract

Preoperative anxiety is prevalent. Patients may require anxiety medications, impacting preoperative teaching and patient satisfaction. No studies were found on the effect of essential oils on anxiety in the preoperative setting. The purpose of this experimental study was to investigate if the essential oil Lavandin is more effective than standard care in reducing preoperative anxiety. A convenience sample of 150 adult patients were randomly assigned to either control (standard care), experimental (standard care plus essential oil Lavandin) or sham (standard care plus jojoba oil) groups. Visual analog scales assessed anxiety on admission and OR transfer. Controlling for baseline anxiety and pain, Lavandin group had significantly lower anxiety on OR transfer suggesting Lavandin is a simple low-risk, cost-effective intervention with potential to improve preoperative outcomes and increase patient satisfaction. Future studies should test the effects of Lavandin into the postoperative phase and in specific populations with documented high anxiety, (*Journal of Perianesthesia Nursing*, 2009).

Reprinted with permission.

Figure 13.2   Exemplar for an unstructured research abstract

Authorship

Early in abstract development, the issue of authorship needs to be considered (Erlen, Siminoff, Sereika, & Sutton, 1997; Salcido, 2002). General guidelines are that an author must make substantive intellectual contributions to a study through all of the following (Gottlieb, 2006):

- Conception and design of the study, or the acquisition/analysis/interpretation of data

- Drafting/revising the manuscript for important intellectual content

- Final approval of the version to be published

Getting Your Abstract Reviewed

Make sure to seek feedback on your abstract before the submission date. Don't forget to spell-check and proofread your abstract for accuracy. Ideal reviewers include your mentor, colleagues who have attended your targeted conference, as well as those who have not been involved with your project (Wood & Morrison, 2011). All these parties will provide valuable feedback from their vantage point.

Poster Presentations

Your poster has been accepted! Compared to podiums, poster presentations are less formal. As a result, poster sessions offer rich, spontaneous discussion and the chance to obtain immediate feedback from viewers who are most interested in your topic (Briggs, 2009; Forsyth, Wright, Scherb, & Gaspar, 2010). An additional advantage of poster sessions is they often allow authors to present research at the earlier, incomplete stage.

Plan for a successful poster session by following established guidelines provided by the conference sponsor. Your acceptance letter will indicate the size for the poster and whether it will be tabletop or wall mounted. Tables are not usually provided with wall-mounted posters. Therefore, plan to fasten an envelope next to your poster if you want to share handouts. Don't forget your business cards as well! Finally, review the conference schedule to determine when poster sessions are held. Most conferences require authors to be present during a dedicated poster session time.

Poster Content

Posters need both well-developed content and visual appeal to attract the audience. Remember the rule of 10s: Average viewers scan posters for 10 seconds from 10 feet away. As a result, you need to be able to present the poster in 10 seconds and viewers should be able to assimilate and discuss the content in less than 10 minutes (Wood & Morrison, 2011).

Break your content into logical segments using the IMRAD method. Decipher the most critical information by asking if it is *nice to know* or *need to know*. Sometimes abstracts are incorporated into posters and appear in the upper-left corner. Briefly draft key points for the introduction, methods, results, and discussion sections (Ellerbee, 2006; Miracle, 2008). Use action verbs whenever possible (Norwood, 2000).

Introduction. In the "Introduction," provide a clear problem statement to communicate the context of your study (Polit & Beck, 2012). Include relevant background information about why you conducted the study. Statistics on the prevalence of the problem (when indicated) also help convey the significance of your topic. At the end of the "Introduction," list the purpose statement and research questions/hypotheses, emphasizing the gap in knowledge your study addressed (Wood and Morrison, 2011).

Methods. The "Methods" section has the following subsections that you need to describe:

1. Design

2. Setting

3. Sample/sample size

4. Interventions tested (intervention studies only)—Describe what was done and in what sequence

5. Instruments/measures

6. Human subject's protection

Results. In the "Results" section, describe the demographic characteristics of your sample, along with the main findings for each research question, even if they're negative. Do not repeat statistical information in text and tables/graphs (Polit & Beck, 2012). Highlight major findings in the narrative, and supplement this text with tables and graphs. For instance, use pie charts for demographic characteristics and/or other variables (Ellerbee, 2006; Miller, 2007). Line graphs are preferred with more than 2 serial data points to convey patterns or trends over time. Conversely, tables are useful with multiple variables/complex data. Relevant statistics (p values, odds ratios, confidence intervals) for key outcomes need to be included (Wood & Morrison, 2011). You can denote statistical significance by boldface, italicization, or contrasting colors (Miller, 2007).

Discussion. Lastly, in the "Discussion" section, compare your main findings with previous research, as well as offer explanations for conflicting evidence (e.g., subject, instrument, statistical method differences). As Wood and Morrison (2011) pointed out, it is essential to avoid overstating your findings. Thus, make sure to not "go beyond your data" by inferring any conclusions that are not supported by the data. After discussing conclusions, end by sharing implications for practice, health care policy, or further research

Poster Format

When you have draft content, it might be helpful to first sketch the poster on paper. Arrange content in a series of three, four, or five columns to facilitate flow (Frantz, 2012). Or, check if your institution has a preferred or required poster template (Wood and Morrison, 2011). As shown in Figure 13.3, posters are typically organized to facilitate a downward newspaper-like reading sequence from left to right. Content should be laid out symmetrically with the most important information centrally located at eye level, and balanced with white space. Therefore, don't overcrowd or clutter the poster with too much or unnecessary information (Ellerbee, 2006; Miracle, 2008).

While content can be developed on individual slides that are mounted on a poster board/wall, most posters created today are one-piece PowerPoint slides that are printed at a large size and laminated. To prepare a poster using this approach, size your PowerPoint document using the following steps:

1. Under Page Setup, look for the Slides Sized For box and select Custom.

2. In the Custom field, specify the width and height.

You can set the page to be as much as half the finished size of the poster and then request the printer to enlarge it (Frantz, 2012) but remember, the final size must meet the maximum dimensions specified by the conference.

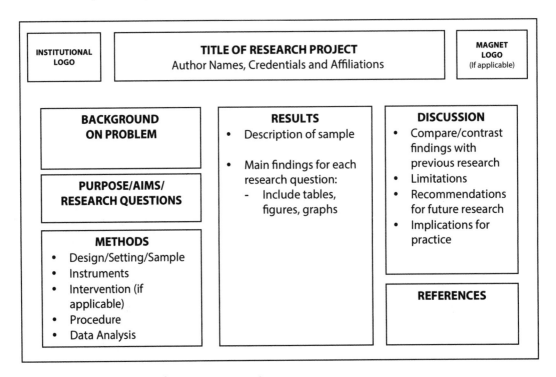

Figure 13.3   Sample format for poster presentation

Using PowerPoint to Create Your Poster

An excellent tutorial of how to construct a poster in PowerPoint is available here: www.nurseweb.ucsf.edu/conf/cripc/posterppt.pdf

Another consideration for size is your budget. Poster printing can cost anywhere from $60 to $200 depending on size (3'×4', 4'×6' or 4'×8').

Poster Design

Consider your topic. Does it conjure up a theme? If so, the theme may lend itself to a particular background, as well as choice of colors and images (Ellerbee, 2006). After you've decided on your background, begin creating the poster by placing the title at the top, followed by author names and affiliations. You should acknowledge funding sources beneath the authors. Use the largest font and a different color to differentiate the title from the body. The title font should be approximately 2" to 3" tall (96 point font or more) (Briggs, 2009; Ellerbee, 2006; Miracle, 2008). Place your organization's logo in the title section after consulting with your marketing department regarding institutional standards for logo use.

From this point, insert text boxes for the remaining sections to tell your research story. Choose headings for the IMRAD sections and boldface them for emphasis. Left justify text for each section. Use short sentences for single ideas, such as your purpose and conclusion statements. Bulleted text helps convey complex content, such as inclusion/exclusion criteria or main findings. Consider your target audience as well; you should avoid highly technical or health care jargon with lay audiences (Forsyth et al., 2010). Use numbers when detailing steps and tables/graphs to condense major findings.

Posters—A Visual Medium

Posters are essentially visual presentations, so try to find ways to show what was done in your project rather than explaining it all with text. Photos of people, action shots, and other illustrations bring your topic to life. For best resolution, photos need 200 to 300 dots per inch (dpi). In general when using photos/illustrations, remember that less is more. Balance the content and visuals with enough white space so your poster is both appealing and easy to read. In one study, visual appeal was found to be more important than content for knowledge transfer (Rowe & Ilic, 2009).

You should also bear in mind the following poster design considerations. First, select two or three colors that work well together for the background. Contrasting colors aid visibility and legibility. You might want to choose colors that accentuate your topic. For instance, red and yellow are stimulating, whereas blue and green are calming (Ellerbee, 2006; Miracle, 2008). As far as text goes, dark lettering on light background (or vice versa) is recommended to create high contrast. All text should have at least a 24 to 36 point font so it can be viewed from 4' to 6'. However, headings should be in a larger font like the title (96 point font or more), boldface, and a different color than the title for emphasis (Briggs, 2009; Ellerbee, 2006; Wood & Morrison, 2011). In general, limit the poster to two types/colors of fonts and stay in the same font family (i.e., sans serif versus serif), as too many fonts/colors can detract from your message (Ellerbee, 2006).

Final Draft and Printing

When you have your poster drafted, print it by checking "scale to fit paper" in the lower part of the Print dialog box. Ask your colleague to critique your poster for honest feedback. What might make total sense to you might be confusing to another eye. Put the poster away for a few days and review the draft with a fresh perspective. Use spell-checker, but also double-check a printed copy for accuracy.

Laminated posters cost considerable money, so you want to make sure there are no typographical errors before you have your poster printed. Allow at least a week turnaround time to print your poster. Large posters can be printed by media departments, local print shops, or office supply/copy centers. If the conference is out of town and you will need to fly to it, purchase a poster tube. Figure 13.4 provides an excellent example of a poster presentation.

Introducing Your Project

Before the conference, map out your primary conversation points. Develop a 10- to 30-second "elevator speech" to introduce your project (Miller, 2007; Wood & Morrison, 2011). Make eye contact as interested colleagues approach your poster but allow them to finish reading before beginning a discussion. Ask viewers if they have questions, and don't forget to follow up with anyone who requested more information after your presentation (Wood & Morrison, 2011).

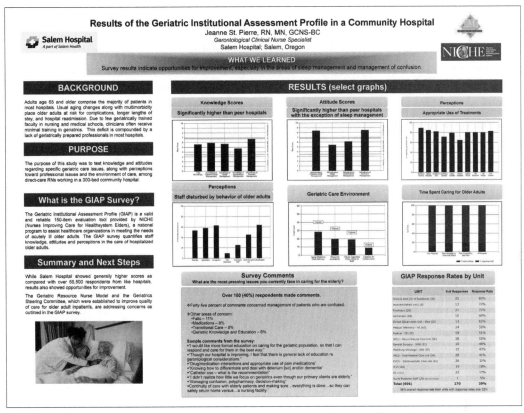

Source: Jeanne St. Pierre, RN, MN, GCNS-BC, Geriatrics Clinical Nurse Specialist, Salem Hospital, Salem, Oregon.
Used with permission of author.

Figure 13.4   Sample poster presentation

Oral (Podium) Presentations

You're a speaker! Podium presentations vary in length but speakers at research conferences are usually allotted 10 to 20 minutes, followed by a short question-and-answer (Q&A). When a series of presentations have been grouped topically as a symposium, the Q&A is generally at the end. Like posters, a main advantage of podium presentations is the opportunity to engage in dialogue with your audience and thus refine your thinking on your study findings. The disadvantage of oral (and poster) presentations is that they reach only very limited audiences (Norwood, 2000).

A main challenge of podium presentations is condensing information in a way that ensures key points are communicated effectively in the time allowed. Again, use IMRAD to create your slide presentation. Draft each section by bulleting key material for the introduction (background), methods (design, sample/setting, instruments, intervention), results (key findings for each research question), and discussion (main conclusions, limitations, implications for practice/further research). Norwood (2000) suggested planning your time for your presentation as follows:

10% Introduction

20% Methods

35% Results

35% Discussion

You should plan for your presentation to cover each slide for 1 to 2 minutes. For example, a 15-minute presentation should have fewer than 15 slides. Slides with text should contain no more than 8 lines, with fewer than 6 words per line. For text slides, black lettering on a white background or white lettering on a blue background are good choices. Just like your poster, don't forget to proofread closely (Norwood, 2000).

After you've developed your slides, practice your presentation to plan comments and time it. Don't memorize your presentation, but familiarize yourself with the content so you sound natural and conversational. Infuse personal experiences and stories about the research process wherever you can to make your presentation more engaging. When you arrive at the conference, it is good advice to check out the room where you will speak to get familiar with the equipment/surroundings (Norwood, 2000). During prime time, expect the moderator to hold up cards to alert you about time left (i.e., 1, 2, 5 minutes). Plan ahead to ensure you can deliver your presentation in the allotted time so you don't have to truncate your speech on the spot. Relax and have fun! It is an honor to have the opportunity to present your research.

The Road to Publication

You've decided to take on the challenge of writing! The major advantages of disseminating your research results through scholarly publication include adding to the body of knowledge on your topic and reaching a considerably larger audience with worldwide accessibility

(Alspach, 2010; Polit & Beck, 2012). Thus, planning is imperative before you dive into your research manuscript. The planning phase involves selecting a journal that reaches your target audience.

Q: *Can I submit my research manuscript to more than one journal at a time?*

A: No. The basic etiquette in science is that authors submit their work to only one journal at a time. Why? Consider this. Let's say you send the manuscript to three journals, and it is accepted by all of them. How would you decide where your work landed because science is only published in one source? As a result, after your manuscript is ready, submit it to your preferred journal. If the manuscript is rejected then you are free to make any necessary changes to increase its chance of acceptance at the journal next on your list.

One great source to learn about professional nursing journals is the Online Nurse Author and Editor website (www.nurseauthoreditor.com/library.asp). At this website, click the Journal Directory tab; you will see an alphabetized list of journals. It may be helpful to peruse journal titles, jotting down those most closely aligned with your topic and nursing specialty. Then go to your library to review them. Careful selection of the journal helps increase your chance of success. Perhaps you want to publish in a general research journal such as *Nursing Research* or a specialty-based research journal such as the *American Journal of Critical Care*. Practice-based journals also publish research, but it's generally in a briefer form.

Journal Guidelines

Learn more about potential journals by downloading author guidelines from www.nurseauthoreditor.com/library.asp. Not only do these guidelines tell you what type of manuscripts journals publish, but also they provide step-by-step instructions on style guidelines such as abstracts, page/word limits, formatting, reference style, or specifications for tables/figures/artwork. Print the author guidelines as they are your roadmap to success!

When you've selected your targeted journals, spend time reviewing several recent issues and finding a model research article that you can emulate. Obviously that author was successful publishing his or her work, so you can use that article to help you keep your eye on the prize.

Just like the poster and podium presentation, use the same title developed for your abstract. If you presented your research in either a poster or podium session, copy and paste the IMRAD content into a Microsoft Word or other document to create an outline and then your first draft. Include key words at the end of your abstract to help readers locate your work when they search for articles on your topic (Polit & Beck, 2012). As Wood and Morrison (2011) suggested the aim is to "double dip" or not reinvent the wheel with each dissemination route. Figure 13.5 provides an example of a research manuscript outline.

Background
Specific Aims
Methods
  Design, Setting and Sample
  Intervention
  Instruments
    Intercultural Development Inventory
    Cultural End-of-Life Care
    Frommelt Attitudes Toward Care of the Dying Scale
    Comfort with End-of-Life Care
Procedure
Results
  Description of the Sample
  Cultural Competence
  Knowledge, Attitudes, Comfort and Satisfaction
  Associations Between Staff Characteristics and Knowledge/Attitudes
Discussion
  Limitations
  Recommendations for Research
Implications for Practice

Figure 13.5   Sample manuscript outline

Learning How to Write for Publication

We recommend the following thorough guides for mastering the content and process of publishing research:

- *Writing for Publication in Nursing* (Oermann & Hays, 2010)

- *Anatomy of Writing for Publication for Nurses* (Saver, 2011)

- *Nursing Research: Generating and Assessing Evidence for Nursing Practice* (Polit & Beck, 2012)

We cannot emphasize enough our recommendation that you seek advice of a colleague who has successfully published research. A writing mentor can assist you in the overlapping phases of writing (Oermann & Hays, 2010). Your mentor will have tips to help you overcome "writer's block," a term that collectively refers to barriers that get in the way of writing. These barriers are different for each author. When you've completed your first draft, Alspach (2010) advised authors to solicit feedback from colleagues who are either experienced and skilled in writing for publication, readers of the journal you have chosen, as well as those not familiar with your project. These reviews will provide a diversity of feedback that undoubtedly will enrich your manuscript.

After you've completed your final edits, it is time to submit your manuscript to your selected journal. Your manuscript will be blinded and then assigned to a panel of reviewers with content expertise in your topic. These reviewers will provide a recommendation to the editor on whether your manuscript should be accepted, revised, or rejected. If at first you don't succeed, learn from the critiques and try again! It is quite rare to have a manuscript accepted with no changes on the first try. So if your manuscript is not outright rejected, expect the editor to ask if you are willing to revise and resubmit your manuscript. Novice authors may need to make multiple attempts to be successful, so draw on the support and counsel of your writing mentor.

Try It Now!

Practice improving the following abstract titles:

- A Randomized Controlled Trial Investigating the Effects of Palliative Care Teams on Quality of Life and Various Symptoms such as Pain, Nausea, Insomnia, and Anxiety in a Large Midwestern Tertiary Medical Center

- Handwashing in Health Care

- A Study of Medication Adherence in Elderly People Who Are Residents in Long-Term Care Facilities and How Medication Management Is a Contributing Factor

- Sepsis Bundles

References

Alspach, G. (2010). Converting presentations into journal articles: A guide for nurses. *Critical Care Nurse*, *30*(2), 8–15.

Braden, B., Reichow, S., & Halm, M. (2009). The use of the essential oil Lavandin to reduce preoperative anxiety in surgical patients. *Journal of Perianesthesia Nursing*, *24*(6), 348–355.

Briggs, D. (2009). A practical guide to designing a poster for presentation. *Nursing Standard*, *23*(34), 35–39.

Ellerbee, S. (2006). Posters with an artistic flair. *Nurse Educator*, *31*(4), 166–169.

Erlen J., Siminoff, L., Sereika, S., & Sutton, L. (1997). Multiple authorship: Issues and recommendations. *Journal of Professional Nursing*, *13*(4), 262–270.

Forsyth, D., Wright, T., Scherb, C., & Gaspar, P. (2010). Disseminating evidence-based practice projects: Poster design and evaluation. *Clinical Scholars Review*, *3*(1), 14–21.

Frantz, D. (2012). *Poster design using PowerPoint*. Retrieved from www.nurseweb.ucsf.edu/conf/cripc/posterppt.pdf

Gottlieb, L. (2006). ICMJE guidelines of assigning authorship and acknowledging contributions. *CJNR*, *38*(3), 5–8.

Milbrett P., & Halm, M. (2009). Characteristics and predictors of frequent utilization of emergency services. *Journal of Emergency Nursing*, *35*(3), 191–198.

Miller, J. (2007). Preparing and presenting effective research posters. *Health Services Research*, *42*(1), 311–328.

Miracle, V. (2008). Effective poster presentations. *Dimensions Critical Care Nursing*, *27*(3), 122–124.

Norwood, S. (2000). *Research strategies for advanced practice nurses*. Upper Saddle River, NJ: Prentice Hall Health.

Nurse Author and Editor. Journals directory. Retrieved from www.nurseauthoreditor.com/library.asp

Oermann, M., & Hays, J. (2010). *Writing for publication in nursing*. New York: Springer.

Polit, D., & Beck, C. (2012). *Nursing research: Generating and assessing evidence for nursing practice*. Philadelphia: Lippincott.

Rowe, N., & Ilic, D. (2009). What impact do posters have on academic knowledge transfer? A pilot survey on author attitudes and experience. *BMC Medical Education*, *9*, 71.

Salcido, R. (2002). Authorship: An occasional source of wounds. *Advances in Skin & Wound Care*, *15*(5), 198–199.

Saver, C. (2011). *Anatomy of writing for publication for nurses*. Indianapolis, IN: Sigma Theta Tau International.

Wood, G., & Morrison, S. (2011). Writing abstracts and developing posters for national meetings. *J Palliative Medicine*, *4*(3), 353–359.

Important Considerations in Research

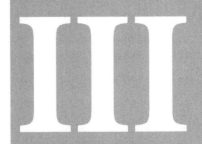

"How do I know what I think
until I see what I write?"

–Anonymous Author

Legal and Ethical Considerations in Research and Publication

14

Shaké Ketefian
Richard W. Redman

WHAT YOU'LL LEARN IN THIS CHAPTER

- Events in history have prompted requirements for human subjects protection.

- Ethical principles guide the protection of humans participating in research, and guidelines are developed based on those principles.

- There are different types of reviews conducted by Institutional Review Boards (IRBs).

As a nurse, you may be leading a research study as the principal investigator (PI), conducting research for the first time with the guidance of a mentor, or helping with a research study that is being conducted in your clinical unit. If you are not the PI, the research investigator may be a nurse or physician colleague, and you might be asked to help with recruitment of patients to participate in the research or collect data from patient records. Although research can provide many exciting opportunities, it also is guided by a number of legal and ethical considerations when human subjects are involved—and all members of the team need to be aware of these considerations. This chapter provides a framework for you to evaluate how to perform your research in an ethical and legal manner.

Protecting Human Subjects: A Modern History

The modern history of human subject protection dates to the era immediately following the Second World War (WWII). In the late 1930s and up to 1945, the Nazi regime in Germany conducted a number of unethical medical experiments on prisoners. These experiments included sterilization, euthanasia, and exposing humans to various environmental conditions such as freezing temperatures and high altitudes. The studies were performed on prisoners who had no opportunity to refuse participation (Grove, Burns, & Gray, 2012).

Following revelations during the Nuremberg trials, during which wanton violations and disrespect of humans were revealed, guidelines were drafted to serve as standards for judging appropriate treatment of human participants in research (The Nuremberg Code, 1947). Subsequently, the World Medical Association developed the *Declaration of Helsinki* (2008; originally adopted in 1964), which has been revised and updated periodically. These two documents have influenced more recent efforts by governments and institutions in their efforts to help guide research in safe, respectful, and dignified ways.

Closer to home in our own country, various abuses of human rights and dignity in research conducted with U.S. government funding came to light. The research in which these abuses occurred became public in the 1960s, 1970s, and in the case of the Tuskegee syphilis studies, over many years starting in the 1930s and lasting until the 1970s. In the syphilis studies, the research traced the natural progression of the disease when untreated, even after it was discovered that the new drug penicillin, developed during WWII, would treat the condition.

In the Tuskegee study, the U.S. Public Health Service conducted a 40-year research project to monitor, but not treat, African-American men who were diagnosed with syphilis. Even when it became evident that the death rate in the men with untreated syphilis was twice as high as that in men who did not have syphilis, the research continued. Information about effective treatments for syphilis was intentionally withheld from the study participants (Grove, Burns, & Gray, 2012).

Collectively, the abuses that were revealed became scandalous, and the U.S. government was moved to address the development of guidelines and procedures to safeguard individuals, and for those most vulnerable, such as children and pregnant women, requiring special attention. Since the very beginning, in 1973–74, guidelines and procedures as highlighted in this chapter have been refined to keep pace with developments in science and societal expectations for accountable governments and accountable science.

As part of the governmental initiative, the U.S. Congress created a national commission to articulate ethical principles to guide the development of procedures to protect human participants in research. The report of the commission came to be known as the *Belmont Report*

(1979); the report has influenced all governmental and institutional procedures that relate to this topic (The National Commission for the Protection of Human Subjects of Biomedical and Behavioral Research, 1979).

Currently, all institutions receiving funding from government agencies and conducting research on human participants have to comply with federal regulations, and institutions have developed their own internal procedures to implement the regulations. The largest agency funding health research within the U.S. government is the National Institutes of Health (NIH), within the Department of Health and Human Services (DHHS. Human subject research is sponsored by other departments of the federal government as well, and researchers are required to follow similar guidelines and regulations.

Obligations When Conducting Research

If you plan to undertake research involving human participants, or subjects, there are two important obligations you must meet:

1. Your first obligation is to the integrity of knowledge, with the goal of generating high-quality science that will contribute to the betterment of society and will serve as a foundation on which others can build.

2. Your second obligation is to treat research participants with dignity, respect, and confidentiality, while assuring that they are safe, fully informed, and are participating voluntarily.

Historically, in western societies the qualities stressed in the preparation and mentoring process of scientists have been honesty, objectivity, openness, trust, and collegiality (Midwest Nursing Research Society [MNRS], 2002). Failures on the part of institutions and research teams in observing these principles have led to the development of rules and regulations that are in place now to enforce these regulations system wide, at the risk of inviting sanctions on both the investigators and institutions for noncompliance.

Ethical Principles

Most guidelines describe ethical principles that underlie various aspects of the mandate to protect research participants from physical, mental, or social harm. However, there are three principles that appear common to all (Belmont Report, 1979):

- Respect for persons

- Beneficence

- Justice

Each of these three principles is briefly described in the following sections.

Respect for Persons

This concept is also referred to in terms of the autonomy of individuals for self-determination and freedom to make judgments as to what will be done to their person. It is also acknowledged that for a variety of reasons, some individuals have diminished autonomy, and, due to their vulnerability, they are entitled to special protections. Vulnerabilities may be due to age, illness, incarceration, or other circumstances (see Chapter 15 for more information on vulnerable populations).

Beneficence

The concept of beneficence refers to the idea of doing good and benefiting individuals. It is expressed in the sense of an obligation to benefit the subjects in the context of research. Other authors, especially philosophers, discuss the principle of nonmaleficence—"do no harm"—as a separate and prior principle that takes precedence to all other principles, including doing good (Beauchamp & Childress, 1994). The idea of doing no harm above all is codified in medical ethics and is implied in nursing's code (ANA, 2001). However, in the Belmont report (1979), nonmaleficence is incorporated under beneficence.

The obligation of beneficence pertains to individuals engaged in research, to the profession to which they belong, professional associations, and to the society at large. The concept of beneficence is used frequently to justify the research enterprise as a whole. More frequently than not, the benefits of research are not likely to accrue to the research participant, but to others at a later time. Given that this is the case, investigators are obligated to be truthful in obtaining informed consent and specifying that while any findings of the research may not benefit them, it is likely to benefit other patients over time (Belmont Report, 1979).

Justice

Theories of justice convey several meanings of the concept; relevant here is one of the meanings of justice, which is *justice as fairness*. Questions such as who participates in research, who carries the burdens, and who benefits from the research are pertinent to justice and fairness. The idea of distribution of benefits and the burdens/risks in society, often referred to as *distributive justice*, is embodied in the second meaning of justice inherent in the use of the concept of justice in this context.

Subjects should not be selected on the basis of their easy availability; instead, they should be selected because they possess characteristics relevant to the purpose of the study. Further, a sense of justice demands that when treatments and therapies become available based on research, all those who need them should be given access. This last point is fraught with controversy and gets us into economic and other arguments that are beyond the scope of this chapter.

An Example of Ethical Principles

An example from a hypothetical research project can help to illustrate how these key ethical principles come into play. Suppose that you are studying an intervention with adolescents in high school and their parents to increase the communication among them around potential or real high-risk behaviors the adolescents may be considering or involved in. Types of behaviors might include use of alcohol or illegal drugs. You are primarily experienced in working with White and African-American families, but the population includes adolescents and their parents from any ethnic or racial group enrolled in the high school. You also recognize that participation is voluntary and is based on full information about the study. Even though the adolescents are not of legal age, you inform them fully about the study and invite their participation (called *assent to participate*). You do the same with the parents, using established informed consent procedures. Using these procedures, it is possible that an adolescent could refuse to participate, even though his or her parents want them to participate in the research.

All three principles are addressed with these study procedures. Respect for persons is addressed through adolescents and parents each having the right and choice to participate or not participate in the study. Because all potential participants participate in assent/consent procedures, they are informed about potential benefits or risks to participation, thus addressing beneficence. And finally, because families from all races and ethnicities have an equal chance to participate in the research, justice is addressed.

Principles Articulated by the Declaration of Helsinki

The *Declaration of Helsinki*, developed by the World Medical Association (WMA, 1964; 2008), provides an extensive list of principles that incorporate general medical ethics as well as those especially relevant for research subject protections. These are generally consistent with the American Nurses Association (ANA) Code (2001) and the MNRS scientific integrity guidelines (2002). The WMA document, which has been revised periodically since its original adoption, covers the following topics, described in more detail in the following sections:

- Considerations in informed consent

- Elements of informed consent

- Documentation of informed consent

- Informed consent and special populations

Considerations in Informed Consent

Respect for persons means a number of important considerations, and it behooves nurse investigators to be mindful of them. Each one of the points identified has to be considered and addressed in view of its relevance to the research project and the nature of the participants being sought. Investigators have to give careful thought to every potential or actual issue that might arise, and the Institutional Review Boards (IRBs) have a responsibility to ascertain and monitor that the matters have been adequately attended to.

The principle of respect for persons means providing truthful information, respecting the subject's voluntary decisions, and maintaining confidentiality of patient information. Where confidentiality cannot be promised, researchers must take steps to assure anonymity. The important distinction between confidentiality and anonymity is that with the latter, data cannot be linked in any way with the identity of the participant, even by the researcher. With confidentiality, data may be separated from the subject's identifying information but the researcher can still link the data to the individual subject.

An example would be with a questionnaire/survey. If you are asked to provide your name and some identifying demographic information, such as age, sex, and race, your answers to the survey items can be linked to you as an individual. If you are not asked to provide any identifying information (such as name, sex, and age) then your responses cannot be linked to you and the data are anonymous.

The principle of justice requires that participants be treated fairly, and that their selection be fair and free of bias. Participants should be protected from discomfort, and they need to be made aware of any discomforts—whether of duration or intensity—and be aware of the potential for any permanent damage that may result. It is incumbent on investigators and reviewers (IRBs) to make assessment of the benefits and risks, and, where possible, maximize the benefits and minimize the risks (Grove, Burns, & Gray, 2012).

 Can I offer incentives to participants in my research project?

 Incentives are payments or gifts offered to research participants as reimbursement for their participation. Incentives are acceptable as long as they are not unduly influential in encouraging someone to participate in a project. For example, offering to pay parking or child care expenses while someone participates in your research project is acceptable because they are viewed as recognition of expenses potential participants might incur for participating in your project. Offering an adolescent $200.00 to complete a questionnaire would be viewed as unduly influential in encouraging participation in the study. Small gift cards would be appropriate. The cost of time and expense incurred for participating in your study have to be balanced against the incentive that you would offer for participating.

Another important matter to consider is the quality of the proposed research. In the early days of the IRBs it was debated whether it is within the purview of IRBs to review the quality of a project, or if the IRBs should solely be concerned with human subject protection and safety. That debate has been resolved in favor of attention to the quality of the proposal as well as human subject protections. It is reasoned that it does not show respect toward research participants to ask them to spend time and effort to participate in projects that deal with insignificant problems, or those that are poorly conceived and designed, where there is no promise of generating science that will have a positive effect on the lives of patients.

Elements of Informed Consent

How do you prepare an informed consent form (ICF)? Many institutions have ICF templates that you must follow; you need to check the availability of this and other relevant resources in your organization. If your employing agency does have a template, you can be assured that it will contain the required elements. Many published books and guidelines discuss this topic and organize it in different ways. The Code of Federal Regulations (45 CFR 46.116, 2010) contains all the regulations for protection of human subjects, including the elements that must be addressed when informing potential subjects about participation in a research project and obtaining their consent to participate in the research. Figure 14.1 presents the elements of informed consent.

A) Providing the prospective participant relevant information:

  1) Describe the projected research.

  2) Describe risks, discomforts, benefits.

  3) In the case of clinical research involving interventions, it may be relevant to describe the alternative interventions available.

  4) Assure subjects of confidentiality and/or anonymity.

  5) If compensation is provided, give information on this. It can be risky to pay participants, due to the possibility that individuals are attracted to participate because of the payment incentive, which might bias or distort study results.

  6) Provide the option to withdraw at any time and assure there will be no negative repercussions.

  7) In instances where some information is being withheld because full information can affect the nature of responses, subjects need to know this in advance, and are entitled to be debriefed following completion of their participation.

  8) Offer to answer any questions.

B) Comprehension of consent information.

  Investigators need to assure that the information provided is understandable to subjects and are given at a level appropriate to them. To this end, many consent documents are prepared in very simplified form. This, however, risks oversimplification, which can mean missing relevant information. As individuals are likely to be at different levels, the offer to answer questions becomes critical. It may be appropriate to ask some questions to determine whether the individual understood the explanation.

C) Competency for consent. There may be individuals who are not capable of understanding the information or to assess risks and benefits; special steps may be indicated in such instances, such as obtaining consent from a legal guardian or next of kin.

D) Consent is given on a voluntary basis. No coercion—subtle or any other kind—is exerted.

Figure 14.1   Elements of informed consent

Documentation of Informed Consent

Written consent is waived at the discretion of the IRB if the risks to subjects are minimal; if there are varying degrees of risk, a written consent form is required. The consent form can be in short form or, if the risks are considerable with unknown outcomes, a full consent, referred to as the *formal written consent document.*

Take, for example, a study that is using a questionnaire to gather data. In this type of research, an information sheet about the research is often included to explain the purposes of the research, its voluntary nature, and how to receive more information about the research if desired. In this case, a written informed consent is generally not required as completion of the questionnaire implies willingness to participate. In fact, it may be preferable to have no identifying information from participants so that names can not be linked with responses. This is an example of a *waiver of informed consent* and only requires a brief information sheet that meets the elements of informed consent. Keep in mind that it is the decision of the IRB to grant the waiver of informed consent.

All other types of research generally require a full consent by the participants, which indicates their explicit agreement to participate and that they have a full understanding of what their participation entails, any risks or benefits involved, and how their data will be maintained. Typically full consent is warranted for this type of research, and the IRB requires a signature from the participants that documents that they have been fully informed of their rights and responsibilities and have consented voluntarily to participate in the research.

Using Templates for Informed Consent Documents

Templates are available to use when developing informed consent documents. Often IRBs provide them to use as guides to ensure that the essential elements of informed consent are addressed. One set of examples for social and behavioral types of research are those provided by the University of Michigan's IRB for Health and Behavioral Sciences (http://www.irb.umich.edu/policies/consent/).

Sample templates for clinical and biomedical research informed consent documents are available here: http://med.umich.edu/irbmed/ict.htm

Consistent with this classification are the levels of review as the outcome of the IRB's work: exempt, expedited, and full reviews. Table 14.1 presents the major types of reviews by an IRB.

Table 14.1   Types of Review by an IRB and Examples of the Nature of the Research

Type of Review	Characteristics and Examples of Research
Exemption from Review	Research may be eligible for exemption according to Federal Regulations if it fits into one of six categories; examples include research involving data that are publicly available or is from a previous research project but all data have been de-identified or research conducted in established or commonly accepted educational settings involving normal educational practices. A complete list of research activities eligible for exemption is provided in 45 CFR 46.101.
Expedited Review	Research that poses no more than minimal risk to research participants and as defined by Federal Regulations falls into one of nine categories that qualify for expedited review; examples include collection of data through noninvasive means or research on individual or group behavior. A complete list of research activities eligible for expedited review is provided in 45 CFR 46.101.
Full IRB Board Review	All research that involves more than minimal risk to research participants or does not fit into one of the specified expedited review categories must be reviewed by the full IRB.

Informed Consent and Special Populations

Individuals/entities from groups such as pregnant women, fetuses, prisoners, human in vitro fertilization, children, or those with mental, cognitive, physical, and other disabilities may have their decision-making competence affected, requiring special consideration and protection. Unequal power relationship between subjects and investigator may create an artificial advantage in favor of the researcher where a faculty member is studying his/her students, for example, and students may not feel sufficiently free to decline to participate for fear of repercussions that might jeopardize their standing as students. Of relevance here is one of the many principles articulated by the Declaration of Helsinki (2008) that addresses special populations:

> "Medical research involving a disadvantaged or vulnerable population or community is only justified if the research is responsive to the health needs and priorities of this population or community and if there is a reasonable likelihood that this population or community stands to benefit from the results of the research."

See Chapter 15 for more detailed information on research with vulnerable populations.

Additional Topics in Scientific Integrity: Authorship

In addition to human subject protection there are other important topics that enhance the integrity and validity of science. This area of study is now known as *scientific integrity*. Other topics are data access and stewardship; considerations in the research process, such as during collection, management, and analysis of data; collaboration within research teams; avoidance of conflict of interest; publication practices that include authorship, peer review, editor and reviewer roles. Here we deal specifically with authorship.

Writing for publication is an important part of the research process; publication of research informs the public and scientific community of the results of your research. If not published, the work does not become known and does not contribute to scientific advancement.

With the trend toward teamwork, it is of critical importance to prospective authors to become aware of who qualifies for authorship. Authorship bestows prestige, brings rewards, and opens new professional, lucrative opportunities. Being listed as author should have clear meaning, both in terms of substantive contribution to the work, as well as assumption of public responsibility for the content of the work.

An author's contribution must be substantive. Substantive contribution means that each individual listed is responsible for two or more aspects of the project: conception and design of the study; execution of the project; analysis and interpretation of data; preparation and revision of the manuscript (MNRS, 2002; For writings that are not based on research, the meaning of these concepts have to be reinterpreted.) As to the order of authorship, there is no clear guidance, with many disciplinary variations. Check with a senior nurse researcher or your mentor for advice.

The MNRS (2002) document provides additional guidance on major elements in authors' responsibilities:

- The project leader assumes overall responsibility for all publications from the project, regardless of whether s/he is listed as an author.

- Team members discuss roles and responsibilities of each person as well as potential authorship and order of authors in advance of preparing manuscripts.

- Position titles should not in and of themselves be the basis for authorship; same with whether a person was paid or not.

- All authors review and approve the manuscript and any revisions.

- Duplicate publications are to be avoided.

This last item is a contentious topic. Some maintain that only one paper should be published from a project; others contend that many projects that are multiyear, multicenter, with large teams are too complex for one paper to do justice. It is also argued that it is possible to write multiple papers without duplication of content. Multiple papers enable team members to report their content more thoroughly, and they can rotate authorship roles among the team (MNRS, 2002). You are advised to read more about this from the references provided at the end of this chapter; also consult with your mentor.

Notes on the Implementation of Policies and Procedures

Institutions such as hospitals or universities where research is conducted have an ethical and legal obligation to ensure that all regulations governing human subjects protections and the ethical conduct of research are adhered to. They are responsible for ensuring that all employees adhere to appropriate policies and procedures that govern research activities so that any research conducted within institutions is in compliance with principles and federal regulations.

The Role of Institutions

Your hospital or institution is responsible to implement governmental regulations on human subject protection, which are now mandatory. They are responsible for creating, training, and maintaining human subject review committees (IRBs) as specified by government regulations, for providing training to all investigators, whether these are full-fledged scientists or trainees/students. In addition, institutions are responsible for monitoring research and investigators on an ongoing basis to ascertain that they are employing procedures as approved by the IRBs.

IRBs are required by the federal government to protect the rights and welfare of human subjects participating in research. The IRB is responsible for reviewing and approving all human research activities to ensure that the universities, hospitals, and their investigators and research teams are compliant with ethical standards, state and federal laws, and institutional policies governing human subject research. The committee is made up of many professionals, including researchers, physicians, nurses, and allied health professionals, and may include faculty, staff, and students from an affiliated university, along with at least one member of the local community, referred to as a member of the lay public or the "community member." The membership collectively must have the experience and expertise necessary to evaluate the proposed research project, as well as have the perspective of regular citizens.

 How do I know if my project requires IRB review?

 Projects meeting the regulatory definition of research with human subjects require either review and approval of an IRB, or a determination that the research is exempt. Not all activities that involve people, their data, or specimens are covered by the regulations governing human subjects research. First, you need to consider if your project is research. Federal regulations define research as systematic investigation, including development, testing, and evaluation that is designed to develop or contribute to generalizable knowledge (45 CFR 46.102, 2010). Research generally does not include activities such as clinical practice. Also, projects for quality assurance or quality improvement (QI) are not research because the intent is to improve local practice or care, not to draw conclusions beyond that practice or program being studied. However, there are some QI activities that may require research. You need to consult with your mentor and your local IRB if you are unsure. Next, you need to consider if your project involves human subjects. Federal regulations define a human subject as a living individual about whom a researcher is obtaining data through intervention or interaction or identifiable private information (45 CFR 46.102, 2010).

Q: *What if I'm not sure that my project is research or requires IRB review?*

A: IRB staff are available to help you determine if your project involves research with human beings. Feel free to contact them to discuss your proposed project and they will help you evaluate how to proceed. This consultation will be very helpful in determining whether you need to seek IRB approval. In any case, you need to obtain IRB approval before any research activities begin on your project.

Professional Societies

Most professions have developed their own codes of ethics; many are now developing their own guidelines for scientific integrity as well. Examples are that of the MNRS that developed its own guidelines in 1996 and issued a revised edition in 2002. The American Psychological Association's *Publication Manual of the APA* (APA, 2009) has provided detailed guidance on these matters for many years and is widely used by students and scholars from several disciplines. The American Medical Association (AMA) provides guidance on human subject protections and other ethical issues involved in research and publication extensively in the *AMA Manual of Style* (2007). Those interested in studying this area in-depth are referred to the *AMA Manual of Style* as a highly useful resource.

Additional Resources

Interested readers can find an extensive list of resources in the professional literature to delve more deeply into these topics. Many of these resources are easily accessed via the Web. Several major resources are presented here as examples:

- The U.S. DHHS has an Office for Human Research Protections (OHRP), which provides leadership in the protection of the rights and well-being of subjects involved in research. Its website provides all the regulations and policies, along with several other educational resources; you can access the site here: http://www.hhs.gov/ohrp/index.html

- NIH, which funds a large portion of the biomedical research in the U.S., also has several resources available for easy access. One example is the website for the Office of Behavioral and Social Sciences Research at NIH (http://obssr.od.nih.gov/index.aspx).

- Many colleges, universities, and academic health centers maintain their own educational programs to educate and certify faculty, students, and staff to ensure that they are knowledgeable about foundations of good research practices when conducting research. An example is the University of Michigan's Program for Education and Evaluation in Responsible Research and Scholarship (http://my.research.umich.edu/peerrs/).

- Although many universities maintain their own training programs to educate and certify faculty, students, and research staff involved in research in their institutions, some do not. Many clinical agencies and hospitals do not have their own training programs. A widely used national resource for training and education in research ethics and human subject requirements is the Collaborative Institutional Training Initiative (CITI), which anyone can participate in. Resources for the CITI program are available here: https://www.citiprogram.org

- Finally, there is variation in requirements for conducting research internationally. Although the ethical principles are universal, the requirements and policies may vary from country to country. A good resource for conducting research in international settings is the "Standards and Operational Guidance for Ethics Review of Health-Related Research with Human Participants" provided by the World Health Organization (WHO; http://whqlibdoc.who.int/publications/2011/9789241502948_eng.pdf).

Navigating the necessary approval for your research proposal and preparing IRB documents can seem overwhelming and daunting at first. But remember that institutions assume overall responsibility for making sure that research being carried out by their members is done with integrity and assures the generation of sound science. This means having in place teaching materials and faculty mentorship, as well as monitoring mechanisms at various levels. Individuals at the highest level of leadership should articulate the importance they place on these matters, and make certain that resources are in place to achieve sound science. Put another way, you should follow the guidelines and protections described in this chapter because it is right to do so, not merely because it is mandatory.

Try It Now!

Find the steps required in your hospital to have a research study approved. For example, is there a nursing research committee that must approve your proposal before you go to the IRB? If so, find out who the chair is and how often the nursing research committee meets. Do you know how to locate the IRB in your institution? Do you know who to contact for questions about submission? How far prior to review does the IRB require your submission? What human subject training in research is required by your institution?

References

American Medical Association. (2007). *The AMA manual of style: A guide for authors and editors* (10th ed.). New York: Oxford University Press.

American Nurses Association. (2001). *Code of ethics with interpretive statements*. Washington, DC: Author. Retrieved from www.ana.org

American Psychological Association. (2009). *Publication manual of the APA* (6th ed.). Washington, D.C.: Author.

Beauchamp, T. L., & Childress, J. F. (1994). *Principles of biomedical ethics* (4th ed.). New York: Oxford University Press.

Collaborative Institutional Training Initiative (CITI). (2013). Retrieved from https://www.citiprogram.org

Grove, S. K., Burns, N., & Gray, J. R. (2012). *The practice of nursing research: Appraisal, synthesis and generation of evidence* (7th ed.). St. Louis, MO: Elsevier/Saunders.

Midwest Nursing Research Society. (1996). *Guidelines for scientific integrity*. Glenview, IL.: Author.

Midwest Nursing Research Society. (2002). *Guidelines for scientific integrity* (2nd ed.). Wheat Ridge, CO: Author.

National Commission for the Protection of Human Subjects of Biomedical and Behavioral Research. (1979). *The Belmont Report: Ethical principles and guidelines for the protection of human subjects of research.* Retrieved from http://www.hhs.gov/ohrp/index.html

Nuremberg Code (1947). Retrieved from http://ohsr.od.nih.gov/nuremberg.php3

University of Michigan. (2013). *Informed consent. Health sciences & behavioral sciences IRB*. Retrieved from http://www.irb.umich.edu/policies/consent/

University of Michigan. (2013). *Program for education and evaluation in responsible research and scholarship (PEERRS)*. Retrieved from http://my.research.umich.edu/peerrs/

University of Michigan. (2013). *Relevant guidance for informed consent. IRB-Med*. Retrieved from http://med.umich.edu/irbmed/ict.htm

U.S. Department of Health & Human Services. (2010) Code of Federal Regulations. Title 45, part 46, Protection of human subjects. (45 CFR 46.116). Retrieved from http://www.hhs.gov/ohrp/humansubjects/guidance/45cfr46.html#46.116

U.S. Department of Health & Human Services. (2010). Code of Federal Regulations. Title 45, part 46, Protection of human subjects. (45 CFR 46.102). Retrieved from http://www.hhs.gov/ohrp/humansubjects/guidance/45cfr46.#46.102

U.S. Department of Health & Human Services. (2013). Office for Human Research Protections (OHR). Retrieved from http://www.hhs.gov/ohrp/index.html

U.S. Department of Health & Human Services. (2013). Office of Behavioral and Social Sciences Research. National Institutes of Health. Retrieved from http://obssr.od.nih.gov/index.aspx

World Health Organization. (2012). *Standards and operational guidance for ethics review of health-related research with human participants.* Retrieved from http://whqlibdoc.who.int/publications/2011/9789241502948_eng.pdf

World Medical Association. (2008). *Declaration of Helsinki – Ethical principles for medical research involving human subjects.* Retrieved from www.wma.net/en/30publications/10policies/b3/index.html

"How far you go in life depends on your being tender with the young, compassionate with the aged, sympathetic with the striving, and tolerant of the weak and strong."

—George Washington Carver

Research With Special Populations

15

Marie Boltz
James E. Galvin

- Nurses are ideally positioned to lead research initiatives with vulnerable persons.

- Nurses need to consider several sources of vulnerability related to health, social, and economic factors when planning research studies.

- Nurses promote equitable access to research opportunities, as well as responsible and respectful research conduct, consistent with federal regulations.

Consider this research study: You plan to pilot a sleep protocol intervention to promote sleep quality and minimize the use of sedative hypnotics on a medical unit. Older adults with cognitive impairment (CI), including dementia, are at particularly high risk for the negative effects of sleep problems, including delirium and falls. This very group has often been excluded from clinical research at your institution because of consent issues. How can you offer the opportunity to persons with CI to be involved in a manner that is ethical and respectful?

The federal regulations of Health and Human Services (HHS; Title 45 Code of Federal Regulations Part 46 [45CFR46], 2005) implement the requirement that researchers take into account the "special problems of research involving vulnerable populations, such as children, prisoners, pregnant women, mentally disabled persons, or economically or educationally disadvantaged persons." Nurses, because of our broad clinical backgrounds, routinely access vulnerable groups in our efforts to better understand and respond to their needs (Beattie & VandenBosch, 2007). Further, our position as trusted health care professionals places us in a unique position to be central advocates for the vulnerable person's engagement in research. The purpose of this chapter is to define vulnerable populations and describe the role of the nurse researcher in promoting equitable access to research opportunities, as well as responsible and respectful research conduct, consistent with federal regulations.

The Concept of Vulnerability

There is no definition of vulnerable subjects per se in the federal regulations other than the identification of the groups currently protected. According to the Council for International Organizations of Medical Sciences (CIOMS, 2002), the chief characteristic of vulnerability is limited capacity or freedom to participate or to decline to participate in research. More specifically, the National Bioethics Advisory Committee (2001) describes six categories of vulnerability, as shown in Table 15.1.

Table 15.1   Vulnerable Populations in Research: An Overview

Vulnerability Category	Description	Population
Cognitive or Communicative Vulnerability		
a. Capacity-related	Lack ability to make decisions	Children Cognitively impaired
b. Situational cognitive	Do not lack capacity but are in situations that do not allow them to exercise that ability	People in stressful emergencies Pregnant women
c. Communicative	Language impairs ability to receive information and make an informed consent	Non-English-speaking subjects
Institutional Vulnerability	Have the capacity to make decisions but are subordinate to formal authority of others	Prisoners Military personnel College students Employees
Deferential Vulnerability	Subordination to an informal authority, based on social inequalities, inequalities related to power and knowledge, subjective inequalities	Gender, race, class Physician/patient relationship Older adults deferring decision to adult children

Vulnerability Category	Description	Population
Medical Vulnerability	Fear and lack of knowledge of medical condition make it difficult to weigh the risks and potential benefits associated with the research.	Subjects who have serious medical conditions for which there is no satisfactory standard treatments
Economic Vulnerability	Disadvantages increase the risk for undue inducements to enroll and threatens the voluntary nature of consent.	Disadvantaged in areas such as income, housing, or health care. (Offers of large amounts of money or access to free health care may induce participation in research against their better judgment.)
Social Vulnerability	Groups that have been stigmatized or stereotyped	Persons with HIV/AIDS Homeless persons

Research in Individuals With Cognitive Impairment

According to the Office for Human Research Protections (OHRP, Department of Health and Human Services) cognitive impairment (CI) is defined as "having either a psychiatric disorder (e.g., psychosis, neurosis, personality or behavior disorders), an organic impairment (e.g., dementia), or a developmental disorder that affects cognitive or emotional functions to the extent that capacity for judgment and reasoning is significantly diminished." Others, including persons under the influence of or dependent on drugs or alcohol, those suffering from degenerative diseases affecting the brain, terminally ill patients, and persons with severely disabling physical handicaps, may also be compromised in their ability to make decisions in their best interests.

Conditions associated with CI cause considerable suffering to affected patients and their families. Consequently, there is a research imperative to identify effective ways to promote brain health, detect CI, and design interventions to promote the coping abilities of persons with CI and their families. Unfortunately, there is a paucity of research in these areas, due in large part to the ethical issues associated with their engagement in research (O'Connor et al., 2007).

Both written consent and verbal consent for participation in research must involve an informed consent process. Informed consent is not merely a signed form; it involves *a process* of education and information exchange that takes place between the researcher and the potential subject. The predominant ethical concern in research involving individuals with CI is that their condition may compromise their capacity to understand the information presented and their ability to make a reasoned decision about participation in research. Additionally, mildly cognitively impaired individuals could be vulnerable to coercion, especially residents of institutions responsible for their total care and treatment. There are basic considerations (Alzheimer's Association, 2004) related to research involving cognitively impaired persons that should guide you:

- CI is *not* always associated with the lack of capacity for informed consent to research (Karlawish, 2003). Excluding persons on the basis of CI alone, whether or not they lack the capacity to consent, is discriminatory and violates the ethical principle of justice (Alzheimer's Association, 2004).

- There are basic conditions that should be met in order to enroll a person with cognitive impairment:

  - The research offers a reasonable prospect of a direct health-related benefit to the person or no more than a minor increment above minimal risk (probability and magnitude of harm or discomfort anticipated in the research are not greater in and of themselves than those ordinarily encountered in daily life), and is likely to yield generalizable knowledge about the participant's disorder or condition.

  - Informed consent for research is provided by someone who, under state or federal law, has the legal authority to make such decisions for the patient.

  - The person with CI assents to participation if capable, or does not dissent.

- If the research involves more than minimal risk (or a minor increase above minimal), the person with CI may be enrolled if he/she has a research advance directive that authorizes a proxy to provide consent for enrollment in research of this kind and the condition causing cognitive impairment is the object of study (Alzheimer's Association, 2004).

The nurse is in a key position to support the ethical involvement of persons with CI in research. The nurse is called upon to act as clinician and advocate to make sure that they are represented in research initiatives, while supporting the person's preferences and well-being.

Steps for the Nurse Researcher to Take

What steps should you take to protect the cognitively impaired patient in research? Important steps include

1. Assessing, that is screening for cognitive impairment and evaluation of capacity to provide informed consent

2. Securing permission and assent

Assessment

When planning a study and applying for Institutional Review Board (IRB) approval, you need to consider whether the population to be studied is at risk for incapacity related to CI. If the study focuses on persons with dementia, the answer is quite obvious. However, other populations have been reported in the literature to have incidence of CI, including patients in intensive care and acutely ill patients in the emergency department, patients with certain psychiatric conditions, residents of nursing homes and assisted living facilities, hospitalized patients with congestive heart failure, patients with AIDS, and persons of very advanced age (Alzheimer's Association, 2004).

Screening for cognitive impairment. When research involves persons at risk for CI, investigators should consider a screening procedure, using a validated tool such as the MINI-COG (Borson, Scanlan, Watanabe, Tu, & Lessig, 2006) or the Montreal Cognitive Assessment, (MoCA; Nasreddine et al., 2005) in their protocol. There are two reasons for this:

1. To identify persons who, because of cognitive impairment, might have difficulty with adherence

2. To identify persons who are unable to consent to the research, thus allowing better targeting of in-depth capacity assessments

The screening itself does not take the place of capacity assessment.

> **Q:** *I work on an ACE (acute care of elders) unit, and I am conducting a study on functional mobility. I would like to observe patients and conduct chart audit. Many of our patients have MINI-COG results that show cognitive impairment. I would like to include all patients age 70 and older in the study, including those with cognitive impairment. Is this possible?*

A: The presence of cognitive impairment, in and of itself, is not a reason to exclude someone. If the person otherwise meets the study's inclusion criteria, you need to consider how to acquire informed consent. The first step in this process is evaluating the person's decision-making ability to make certain that they can understand the study purpose and activities and give consent to participate.

Evaluating decision making. The IRB application should describe how capacity will be assessed and whether a formal tool will be used. The investigator, or IRB-approved designee, at a minimum, must review and discuss the research project, and the consent document, with the potential participant and decide whether he or she is able to describe the nature of the research and participation, the consequences of participation, alternatives to participation (including the choice to not participate), and demonstrate the ability to make a reasoned choice (Alzheimer's Association, 2004). The discussion should include both oral and written description of the research (purpose, procedures, risks, benefits, alternatives), presented sequentially in simple language without jargon. The written material should use a type font and size that is easily readable by older subjects, such as Times New Roman 13 or 14 pt font or Georgia 12 or 13 pt font (National Institute on Aging, 2008).

Investigators may choose to use the MacArthur Competence Assessment Tool for Clinical Research (Carpenter et al., 2000; Karlawish, 2003) to evaluate the patient's capacity to consent. This tool assesses four elements of decisional capacity that are related to the generally applied legal standards for competence to consent to treatment and research. They include the ability to:

- Understand the information relevant to the decision

- Appreciate the information (applying the information to one's own situation)

- Use the information in reasoning

- Express a consistent choice regarding participation (Dunn, Nowrangi, Palmer, Jeste, & Saks, 2006)

A second tool, the Evaluation to Sign Consent, is briefer than the MacArthur Competence Assessment Tool and assesses the patient's alertness/ability to communicate, ability to describe the risks of the study, things that the participant is expected to do, right to refuse, and what the patient would do in the event of distress or discomfort during the study (Resnick et al., 2007).

Q: *I plan to conduct research on transitions of care from the emergency department to the medical-surgical units. I plan to follow patients throughout the course of the hospital stay. Can I just use the Evaluation to Sign Consent without screening for cognitive impairment?*

A: Screening for cognitive impairment in at-risk populations is important to establish baseline cognition and, therefore, detect any subsequent change in cognition. This is important not only to guide clinical management but also to evaluate the person's cognitive ability to continue to provide consent throughout the study.

Permission and Assent

If a potential participant is determined to lack capacity to consent to the research project, the investigator ordinarily must obtain permission from a proxy with both actual capacity and legal authority to give it, as well as assent from the participant. *Assent* is defined as an affirmative agreement to participate in research, which is required by federal and state statutes (Alzheimer's Association, 2004). Most state laws rank the priority level for the participant's legally authorized representative. If a potential proxy is not available at a given priority level, the investigator should seek to identify a proxy from the next level down (Alzheimer's Association, 2004):

1. Legal guardian.

2. Proxy (research agent) named in the participant's research-specific advance directive.

3. Proxy (health care agent) named in an advance directive or durable power of attorney for health care.

4. Family member or other surrogate identified by the state law on health care decisions. This is often the person who provides permission, usually a spouse, child, caregiver, or other trusted individual, for decisions of everyday life or medical care.

Securing permission from the proxy. The Alzheimer's Association (2004) recommends that the consent include instructions to the proxy to base his or her decisions on the participant's expressed wishes or, in the absence of expressed wishes, what the participant would have desired in light of his or her prognosis, values, and beliefs. If the participant's wishes are unknown and cannot be inferred, the decision should be based on the participant's best interests. The instructions should also include a statement that the proxy should consider how much the subject would have granted the proxy leeway or freedom to choose for the subject.

Assent from the participant. If the participant is capable of providing an affirmative agreement to participate, the participant should be informed in the presence of the proxy that he or she is about to be enrolled in a research study. The procedures, risks, benefits, and alternatives involved should be explained in a simple fashion. The participant should then be asked if he or she agrees to be in the research study, and the response should be recorded. If the participant is incapable of providing affirmative agreement to participate, then assent (or dissent) should be judged behaviorally based on cooperativeness with study procedures (e.g., does he or she refuse to take part in evaluation or planned intervention, even after appropriate communication techniques are employed ?). Dissent for any study-related procedure should be respected, and consistent dissent may be a basis for removal from the research study.

Changes in capacity to consent. If the participant is enrolled in the study through proxy permission and then at any time regains the capacity to provide permission, the investigator must obtain the participant's informed consent for continued participation in the research. If a participant who gave his/her own consent appears to lose capacity during the study, the investigator must formally assess the participant's capacity to consent, and if capacity is impaired, obtain permission for further research participation from a proxy.

Q: *I have a patient who consented to participate in a fall prevention study but then developed cognitive changes after hip surgery, with new-onset disorientation, lethargy, and decreased attention span. He now has an abnormal MINI-COG and confusion assessment method consistent with a postoperative delirium. Do I need to drop him from the study?*

A: Not necessarily. You need informed consent from him or his proxy to continue his participation. First, determine his decision-making capacity, using a tool such as the Evaluation to Sign Consent tool. If he is able to answer all questions correctly and agrees to continue in the study, then this is considered continued informed consent. If he is not able to answer your questions about his understanding of the study, but assents to the study, the next step would be to acquire informed, signed consent from his legally authorized surrogate decision-maker

(legal guardian, research agent named in his advanced
directive, health care proxy, or family member or other
surrogate identified by the state law on health care decisions).
You should continue to evaluate the patient's assent, cognition,
and capacity for consent, and seek his consent when/if he is able
to do so.

The Child as a Vulnerable Subject

Federal regulations (45 CFR 46, 2005) state, "'Children' are persons who have not attained
the legal age for consent to treatments or procedures involved in the research, under the
applicable law of the jurisdiction in which the research will be conducted." Who qualifies as a
"child," therefore depends on local laws for consent (typically age 18 or age 21).

Permission Requirements for Research With Children.

Federal regulations classify permissible research involving children into four categories.
These categories are based on the degree of risk and type of individual subjects (45 CFR
46.405-407, [2005]; 21 CFR 50.51-54, [2013]). These categories are described in relation to
"minimal risk."

1. *Research not involving greater than minimal risk.* An example includes a nurse-led,
   interdisciplinary, culturally sensitive oral health educational program for preschool
   age children. In addition to assessing the knowledge of parents, the oral health and
   hygiene of the child will be assessed on an ongoing basis for several months. This
   requires permission from at least one parent (or guardian).

2. *Research involving greater than minimal risk but presenting the prospect of direct benefit
   to the individual subjects* requires permission from at least one parent (or guardian).
   An example includes a clinical trial of a chemotherapeutic agent.

3. *Research that involves more than minimal risk and presents the prospect of no direct benefit to individual subjects, but generalizable knowledge (societal benefit)* about the subject's disorder, condition, or situation requires permission from both parents, unless
   one parent is deceased, unknown, incompetent, or not reasonably available, or when
   only one parent has legal responsibility for the care and custody of the child. If these
   circumstances are present, you should document this in the subject's research record.
   An example of this research is an efficacy evaluation of an invasive diagnostic procedure that may also inform the individual patient's treatment options.

4. *Research not otherwise approvable which presents an opportunity to understand, prevent, or alleviate a serious problem affecting the health or welfare of children* requires the same permission as category 3.

In the cases where two parents are available to give permission, they must both agree on allowing their child to participate in the study. In all categories of research, assent of the child (if child is 7 years of age or older) is required.

Child Assent

In most cases, assent must be documented in writing if the subjects are at least seven years old. The institution's IRB may require assent from children younger than seven if they are likely to comprehend and appreciate what it would mean to volunteer to participate in a given protocol.

When developing an assent form, consider the educational level and maturity level of the youngest potential subject in the age range. Large font-size type, simple schema, and pictures help promote the child's understanding of the text. If there is a wide age range of children to be involved, two different assent forms at different reading comprehension levels (e.g., one assent form written for young children ages 7–12 years old and one assent form written for minors ages 13–17 years old). You can also develop a joint assent/permission consent form and obtain the signatures of the minor and parent(s) or guardian(s) on one document for the age group of children 13–17 years of age (Kodish, 2003).

An assent form should contain date and signature lines for the child, a witness, and an investigator. According to Ross (2006), the following elements should be in the assent form: what the study is about, why the child is eligible to participate for the study, what procedures will be performed, potential risks and discomforts to the child, potential benefits to the child and society, a statement that the child can choose whether to participate and may withdraw at any time without negative consequences, an invitation to ask questions any time, and names and phone numbers of whom to contact with questions.

Sensitive matters involving children. The permission and/or assent form should describe plans for disclosure or nondisclosure of sensitive issues such as sexual activity, sexually transmitted diseases (STDs), use of illegal substances, and child abuse. Ethical and legal obligations apply whenever child abuse is discovered. You should be aware that, in most cases, the same mandatory reporting laws apply in research settings as in clinical settings. Even if the mandated reporter status is not clear, the researcher can make a voluntary report to the appropriate agency.

Enrolling children in long-term studies. If the study continues past the point at which the subject is no longer considered a minor, "reconsenting" is usually required, unless a review of records or examination of biological specimens are the only continuing study activities. In these cases, the original consent may suffice.

Q: *I plan to conduct a research study on dyads comprised of mothers and their diabetic children, ages 8–14, to take part in an educational program to support healthy food choices, exercise, and health monitoring. Who should give consent for the study?*

A: Consent from the parents will be required for their own involvement in the study, as well as the participation of the minor (a person under age 18). Assent is also required from the minor. You should plan to explain the study to the parents and children. Because there is a wide variation in the age and reading levels, develop one assent form written for the younger children (ages 8–11) and one for the children age 12 and older. For the children ages 12–14 years of age, you can use a joint assent/permission consent form and obtain the signatures of the minor and parent(s) or guardian(s) on one document.

Prisoners as Vulnerable Subjects

In response to reports of prisoner abuse, federal regulations have protected incarcerated persons involved in federally funded research (45CFR46, Subpart B, 2005) since 1978. Prior to that time the incarcerated arguably carried a heavier burden of research risk than the general population (Beattie & VandenBosch, 2007). Approximately 90 percent of all pharmaceutical research was conducted on prisoners, as was research involving the development of diet drinks, detergents, dioxin, and chemical warfare agents (Gostin, 2007).

As a group, incarcerated persons present with a multitude of acute and chronic physical and mental health care needs; they are subject to discrimination, stigmatization, and marginalization; and they often experience multiple or overlapping vulnerabilities (Peternel-Taylor, 2005). To protect this study population, federal regulations stipulate that the only studies that may use prisoners are those with an independent and valid reason for involving them, specifically research that is focused on improving the environments of correctional settings, improving rehabilitation, and increasing understanding of diseases common in the prisoner population, such as HIV/AIDS, mental illness, substance abuse, and hepatitis (Beattie & VandenBosch, 2007; Brewer-Smyth, 2008).

Staff and Students as Subjects

If you include peers, students, and subordinates (including employees of the involved institution) in research you are urged to exercise great caution to avoid even the appearance of pressuring or coercing potential subjects into enrollment or continued participation (Beattie & VandenBosch, 2007). In addition, you should guard against the potential for compromised objectivity when including these subjects in a study. The protocol should delineate your plan to maintain confidentiality, including not disclosing study results and/or performance to those in position of authority.

Q: *I plan to evaluate the work/home stressors of females who work in nursing for my Capstone project. I'm the director of Medical Nursing at a large hospital, so I plan to survey the staff there. One of my classmates mentioned that staff might be uncomfortable with this. Should I be concerned?*

A: Your classmate is correct in that you need to make sure that staff do not feel coerced into participating or that, if they do participate, there are methods in place to ensure confidentiality. Ideally, the study would be conducted on alternate units, not under your supervision. If not possible or feasible, then you should be clear in the study information that involvement in the study is voluntary and that there are no consequences of participating or not participating. Methods of safeguarding confidentiality would include not linking names and identifiers to responses and reporting findings in aggregate form (as opposed to ways that identify the survey respondents).

Working With Vulnerable Populations: Additional Considerations for the Nurse Researcher

In addition to being aware of the regulations related to working with vulnerable populations, Beattie and VandenBosch (2007) recommend that you consider some practical and ethical issues. They advise the investigator know the population to be studied, in order to cultivate a climate of respect and openness when partnering with them. It is also important to know of other research conducted within the population in order to build upon the current knowledge. They also recommend that you develop a strong relationship with a member or members of the vulnerable group who can act as a guide to support the researcher's understanding of population norms. An example is a nurse researcher whose research focused on persons with HIV and thus included affected persons on her research advisory panel.

One of the most important considerations for the nurse researcher is the moral imperative to conduct research with vulnerable populations. In the past, researchers have avoided working with vulnerable populations, such as persons with HIV or dementia, or individuals who were economically deprived, believing it to be unethical and too difficult to do (Alexander, 2010). There is significant evidence in existing literature that, not only is research among vulnerable populations unlikely to result in harm, but there are often benefits to be gained by both participants and researchers (Wilson & Neville, 2009). In addition to the general benefits of increased knowledge and improved interventions, participants might benefit from the enhanced knowledge, sense of empowerment, and opportunity to contribute to society (Alexander, 2010).

Try It Now!

You are piloting a new tool to measure the effects of supplementing analgesics with a brief guided imagery activity in postoperative orthopedic patients. The outcome measures include pain levels, blood pressure, and heart rate. A previously mentally intact older adult had consented to participate. Two days after enrollment, the patient becomes confused, demonstrating a delirium, evident on his cognitive evaluation (abnormal MINI-COG and positive CAM). Describe how you should proceed with the study, given his change in mentation. What tools could you use to reassess capacity to consent? What additional steps would you need to take to proceed with this participant in your research study?

References

Alexander, S. J. (2010). "As long as it helps somebody": Why vulnerable people participate in research. *International Journal of Palliative Nursing, 16*(4), 174–179.

Alzheimer's Association. (2004). Research consent for cognitively impaired adults: Recommendations for institutional review boards and investigators. *Alzheimer Disease and Associated Disorders, 18*(3), 171–175.

Beattie, E. R. A., & VandenBosch, T. M. (2007). The concept of vulnerability and the protection of human subjects of research. *Research and Theory for Nursing Practice: An International Journal, 21*(3), 156-173.

Borson, S., Scanlan, J. M., Watanabe, J., Tu, S. P., & Lessig, M. (2006). Improving identification of cognitive impairment in primary care. *International Journal of Geriatric Psychiatry, 21*(4), 349–355.

Brewer-Smyth, K. (2008). Ethical, regulatory, and investigator considerations in prison research. *ANS. Advances in Nursing Science, 31*(2), 119–127.

Carpenter, W. T., Gold, J. M., Lahti, A. C., Queern, C. A., Conley, R. R., & Appelbaum, P. S. (2000). Decisional capacity for informed consent in schizophrenia research. *Archivses of General Psychiatry, 57*(6), 533–538.

Council for International Organizations of Medical Sciences (CIOMS). (2002). International ethical guidelines for biomedical research involving human subjects. *Bulletin of Medical Ethics, 182,* 17–23.

Dunn, L. B., Nowrangi, M. A., Palmer, B. W., Jeste, D. V., & Saks, E. R. (2006). Assessing decisional capacity for clinical research or treatment: A review of instruments. *American Journal of Psychiatry, 163*(8), 1323–1334.

Gostin, L. O. (2007). Human subject research on prisoners. *Georgetown Law Faculty Blog.* Retrieved from http://gulcfac.typepad.com/georgetown_university_law/2006/09/human_subject_r.html

Karlawish, J. H. T. (2003). Research involving cognitively impaired adults. *New England Journal of Medicine, 348*(14), 1389–1392.

Kodish, E. (2003). Informed consent for pediatric research: Is it really possible? *Journal of Pediatrics, 142*(2), 89–90.

Nasreddine, Z. S., Phillips, N. A., Bédirian, V., Charbonneau, S., Whitehead, V., Collin, I., & Chertkow, H. (2005). The Montreal Cognitive Assessment, MoCA: A brief screening tool for mild cognitive impairment. *JAGS, 53*(4), 695–699.

National Bioethics Advisory Commission. (2001). Ethical and policy issues in research involving human participants. Retrieved from http://bioethics.georgetown.edu/nbac/human/oversumm.html

National Institute on Aging. (2008). Making your printed health materials senior friendly. Retrieved from http://www.nia.nih.gov/health/publication/making-your-printed-health-materials-senior-friendly

O'Connor, D., Phinney, A., Smith, A., Small, J., Purves, B., Perry, J.,& Beattie, L. (2007). Personhood in dementia care: Developing a research agenda for broadening the vision. *Dementia, 6*(1), 121.

Office for Human Research Protections (OHRP), Department of Health and Human Services. The IRB guidebook. Retrieved from http://www.hhs.gov/ohrp/archive/irb/irb_chapter6.htm#g5

Peternel-Taylor, C. A. (2005). Conceptualizing nursing research with offenders: Another look at vulnerability. *International Journal of Psychiatry, 28*(4), 348–359.

QuotationsBook. (n.d.). Retrieved from http://quotationsbook.com/quote/35944/#sthash.4UuexCmb.dpbs

Resnick, B., Gruber-Baldini, A., Pretzer-Aboff, I., Galik, E., Buie, V. C., Russ, K., & Zimmerman, S. (2007). Reliability and validity of the evaluation to sign consent measure. *Gerontologist, 47*(1) 69.

Ross, L. F. (2006). *Children in medical research.* New York: Oxford University Press.

U.S. Department of Health and Human Services Code of Federal Regulations. Title 45, part 46, Protection of human subjects. (45 CFR 46.405-407). (2005). Retrieved from http://www.hhs.gov/ohrp/humansubjects/guidance/45cfr46.html

U.S. Department of Health and Human Services Food and Drug Administration Code of Federal Regulations. Title 21, part 50. (21 CFR 50.51-54). (2013, April 1). Protection of Human Subjects. Retrieved from http://www.accessdata.fda.gov/scripts/cdrh/cfdocs/cfcfr/CFRSearch.cfm

Wilson, D., & Neville, S. (2009). Culturally safe research with vulnerable populations. *Contemporary Nurse, 33* (1), 69–79.

> *"Money, by itself, does not make good research.*
> *Good researchers do that."*
>
> –Lawrence Locke, Waneen Spirduso, and Stephen Silverman

Funding Your Study

Claudia DiSabatino Smith

16

After you have developed a solid, feasible research study, it is time to consider how the proposed study will be funded. Most contemporary hospitals and/or clinical agencies do not include money for nursing research studies in their annual operating budgets. Therefore, it is important for you and your research team to spend time designing a study that is not only feasible for you to conduct in your setting, but one that is financially feasible. This chapter explains how to estimate costs associated with conducting your study and how to develop an effective budget to cover those costs. It also suggests where to look for available money and provides tips for increasing your success in securing the funding. Some basic principles of grantsmanship will be presented, along with a list of possible research funding sources.

Why Should I Look for Funding?

Securing research funding may contribute to the increased quality and rigor of your research study overall. Research funding enables researchers to design studies with larger sample sizes that produce stronger, more scientific results. With funding, you are more likely to be able to:

- Enroll a larger sample of similar participants to increase the likelihood that each research participant has the same probability of being selected, therefore reducing sample bias

WHAT YOU'LL LEARN IN THIS CHAPTER

- Before you seek funding, take the time to estimate your actual costs; do not underestimate and do not overestimate.

- After estimating your study costs, create a formal study budget that matches your potential funder's guidelines.

- For nurses who develop strong research studies, many sources of public and private funding are available.

- Use valid and reliable instruments in measuring outcomes

- Enroll and study participants over a longer period of time, which may contribute to sustainability of the proposed intervention

- Employ technical specialists to increase the quality of the study

- Travel to acquire special skills

- Budget for more than minimal equipment, materials, and supplies to enable the research team to focus on conducting the research and not on dwindling materials required for the research

Another reason for securing research funding is that it helps you to establish a track record of studies for which you have received funding. This is important as you look for larger amounts of funding when designing larger, more complicated studies, or when you are seeking federal grant funding.

Q: *I have developed a qualitative study in which I am going to conduct group interviews with registered nurses to identify attributes of clinical credibility. I am working full time and plan to fund the study out of my pocket. A colleague has suggested that I submit a small grant application to the Texas Nurses Association to fund the study. Why should I seek funding if I can afford to pay for the study myself?*

A: If you are eligible for a small grant, there are several reasons to apply for it: The process of submitting a grant affords the researcher an opportunity to practice the skills of grantsmanship; it helps to establish a track record for the researcher that is invaluable when requesting larger sums of money; it also provides the researcher with money so as to offer light refreshments to study participants, or participation incentives such as a $25 gift card or free parking.

Consider Your Research Proposal First

Although it is important to consider available funding, it is also important to remember that money does not make good research. Good researchers make good research (Locke et al., 2000). A strong, solid research proposal will go far in helping to secure the necessary funding.

The amount of money available to a researcher also influences the way that a problem is studied; in fact, it may directly affect the study design. In a recent hospital-based research study (Grami and Smith, unpublished), for example, data was collected by a research coordinator assistant who retrieved patient information that was documented in the medical record by the nursing staff. The study team soon recognized that if the team collected data by directly querying patients and taking their vital signs then there would be more accurate data and less missing data. However, this small change in the data collection method would significantly increase the cost of the study. It would not only require an increase in the number of data collectors, but also an increase in the skill level required, and in the amount of time required for data collection. In this example, the availability of research funding would enable the researcher to increase study personnel costs in an effort to increase the accuracy of the data and decrease the amount of missing data. This is just one example that demonstrates the effect that changes in the study design have on study costs.

The Impact of Funding on Study Design

Research projects may range in cost from a few hundred dollars to hundreds of thousands of dollars for complex study designs. Therefore, it is not unusual to make modifications to an early draft of a research proposal in an effort to develop a financially feasible study. And in some cases, great research ideas may be abandoned altogether due to the expense associated with conducting the proposed study.

Operationalizing a Research Study: The First Step in Estimating Costs

After you have finalized your research study, it is important to operationalize it by crafting a protocol that details each step required to conduct the study. Although protocols are more closely associated with quantitative research studies, they can be used to estimate costs for both quantitative and qualitative studies. The detailed step-by-step protocol then serves as a research manual that guides research team members in the conduct of the study. Table 16.1 demonstrates the difference between "obtaining informed consent" as it appears in a research study proposal and "obtaining informed consent" as it is operationalized in a research protocol.

Table 16.1   Research Study Proposal Versus Research Protocol

Research Study Proposal	The principal investigator or a member of the research team will explain the study, answer questions, and secure informed consent prior to enrolling participants into the study.
Research Protocol	Research team members will recruit study participants.

Research Protocol (continued)

Introducing the Study

Patients *must have completed* their preoperative assessment and preparation prior to enrollment in the music intervention study.

I.   The principal investigator (PI)/ research team member will identify potential participants by reviewing the surgery schedule on the day prior to or on the morning of surgery.

II.   Once admitted to Day Surgery, preoperative preparation is completely done, and patient has been noted on the STAT Com as ready, a member of the research team will interview identified patients to determine whether they are suitable for inclusion or interested in participating in the study (see Inclusions and Exclusions).

III. A team member will introduce the study, "An Exploration of the Duration of Self-selected Music in Reducing Preoperative Anxiety," (Mc Clurkin, unpublished) to qualified participants. The study will be explained and participants will be given an opportunity to ask questions, after which they will be asked to give informed consent. (See consent form.)

Consenting

Informed consent (See form A.)

a.   The principal investigator (PI)/research team member will provide informed consent to the study participant.

b.   Study participant will sign consent and the assigned participant's number will be placed on the upper-right side of the front page.

c.   A copy of the signed consent will be given to the patient for her records.

d.   A copy of the signed consent will be stapled to other documents belonging to the study participant and placed in an envelope.

e.   Tell participants that they can withdraw anytime during the study.

IV.   All study participants will be asked to complete a demographic questionnaire (see Form B – demographic information form).

V.   All study participants will be asked to complete the State Trait Anxiety Inventory (STAI) form (see Form C – sample STAI) prior to the intervention. Please make sure to encourage participants to answer the questionnaire according to "how they feel."

The protocol provides rich detail and enables the researcher to determine actual processes, personnel, and time required to realistically conduct the research. A protocol forces the researcher to move from study conceptualization to concrete planning, as shown in Table 16.1. This is particularly important in interventional quantitative research studies, but is also helpful for any researcher who is estimating costs. After you have operationalized your research proposal, it is time to estimate your study costs.

Estimating Study Costs

Research study costs emerge from your study protocol. Many universities and some hospitals have research centers with an administrator who is skilled in developing budgets for research grant proposals. If such a person is available to you at your institution, it might be wise to seek their assistance in developing your study budget. However, if you are like many of us who work at institutions who lack such formal assistance, let common sense be your guide. Cost categories are generally similar among quantitative studies, although they vary from those commonly found in qualitative studies.

Q: *How do the cost categories of a budget for a quantitative study differ from those of a qualitative study?*

A: In a quantitative study, budgeted items include items such as fees to use copyrighted measurement instruments and pay for a statistician, as well as expenses for paper, postage, envelopes, research assistant hours, phlebotomy equipment, disposable gloves, gift cards that are used as participant incentives, and lab fees. The budget items in a qualitative study include such items as two digital recorders, transcriptionist fees, computer software program, paper, envelopes, refreshments, and gift cards that are used as participant incentives.

Common cost categories include things such as:

- Required number and skill of personnel (registered nurse [RN], research coordinator assistant, data entry clerk)

- Hourly rate of compensation for personnel

- Average time per participant (to enroll study participants, to carry out an intervention [or interview], to collect data, to enter data)

- Average time required for the entire sample size

- Office supplies (paper, pens, printer ink, postage stamps, envelopes, clip boards, photocopying)

- Medical supplies (gloves, tape, blood tubes)

- Incentives (gift cards, thank-you cards, meal tickets)

- Data collection and analysis (cost to use measurement instruments, statistician fees, transcription fees)

- Travel (registration, airfare, taxi, hotel)

- Miscellaneous (Institutional Review Board fee, presentation poster)

Let's estimate the cost of administering a paper-and-pencil survey to study participants in the control group of a quantitative study in which survey responses are placed in a locked box on a patient care unit as described in Figure 16.1 on the opposite page.

Q: *I've been preparing an estimate of my study costs, but they seem too low. Should I pad my study costs to compensate for unexpected expenses?*

A: It is important to avoid both under- or overestimating. Underestimating will cause you to come up short of cash during the course of the study, which could jeopardize the completion of the study if you are not able to secure additional funding. Overestimating may spoil your chances for securing a grant award.

Developing the Study Budget

After you have estimated the study costs for each segment of the study, then transfer the cost estimations into the budget format required by the funding agency. If the funding agency does not provide a formatted budget document, you should create a clear but meaningful table within which to display the budget. The budget is a working document that provides you with expense parameters that, when maintained, will ensure sufficient funds to complete the project.

Q: *The agency I'm requesting funding from doesn't require a specific format for my budget? What should I do?*

A: If the funding agency does not require a specific format, then you may develop the budget by combining the cost estimates for each segment of the study.

Cost Estimate		
Item: Paper Surveys	**Cost Calculation**	**Cost**
1. The survey instrument is in the public domain; does not require payment for its use.	$0.00	$0.00
2. The survey is three pages long and will be printed on blue paper for a sample size of 100. We will make double-sided copies, which will require two pages for each participant, or a total of 200 sheets of blue paper. It is wise to add about 10% additional paper to compensate for printing errors, participants who lose the survey, and participants who drop out of the study (participant attrition). This will increase the total number of sheets of blue paper to 220. One package of blue paper contains 250 sheets and costs $5.45.	2pg x 100 =200 200 x 10% = 20 200+20= 220 250 pgs/ package 250 pgs = $5.45	$5.45
3. Each completed survey will be placed in a legal-size envelope and sealed before returning it to the investigator. Fifty legal size envelopes are in one package and cost $6.95 per package. We will need two packages.	100 surveys = 100 envelopes 50 envelopes/ package 50 envelopes = $6.95 2 x $6.95 = $13.90	$13.90
4. Photocopying surveys and envelopes	220 x $0.10 = $22.00 100 x $0.10 = $11.00	$33.00
	Total	$99.35

Figure 16.1   Estimating costs

As you are estimating your costs, it is important to carefully read the potential funder's guidelines for grant submission. The guidelines specify costs that are covered by the grant, as well as those that aren't covered. Many professional organizations do not cover indirect costs. Indirect costs are not directly related to the conduct of the study, but are associated with institutional overhead such as office space, lights, pagers, and telephones. See Figure 16.2 for an example of a quantitative research budget that was submitted to a professional organization for funding.

Delirium Study Budget 2011				
PERSONNEL (Unless restricted by grant requirements)				
Item #	Position/Title Data Management	Total Number of Hours	Hourly Rate	Total
1	Staff RN Data Collector	15 hours per day x 16 weeks 30 minutes per patient; ADC=30 5 hours per unit/day	$35 per hour $525 x 112 days	$58,800.00
2	Staff training 2 hours per RN staff member 7S1/2 = 55 RNs 7S3 = 26 RNs	81 RNs at their base rate (base rate is different for each nurse; Average is $35 hr.	$70 per staff (81 staff members)	$5,670.00
3	Development of education tools	6 hours at base rate	6 x $35 =	$210.00
4	Statistician	40 hours	40 x $75 =	$ 3000.00
Section Total				**$67,680.00**

CONSUMABLE SUPPLIES (Include only if not provided by institution)					
Item #	Supplies	Costs	% Tax	Tax	Total
4	Printing supplies/paper	2 boxes (28.10 per box)	N/A		$56.20
Section Total					**$56.20**

PERMANENT EQUIPMENT (To be kept by institution after study is done)					
Item #	Technical/Equipment	Costs	% Tax	Tax	Total
6	Projector for training sessions; laptop computer	$350.00 $500.00			$850.00
Section Total					**$850.00**
TRAVEL (Related only to conduct of study)					
Item #	Mileage/Gas/Parking Fees/Etc.	Costs	% Tax	Tax	Total
	No mileage needs identified				$0.00
OTHER COSTS					
Item #	Miscellaneous Costs	Costs	% Tax	Tax	Total
7	Present findings at professional conference 2012; Cost of hotel, airfare, registration	Hotel 3d x 0 $250/d, Air $450, Reg. $500		0	$1,700.00
Section Total					
				Sub Total	$1700.00
% Indirect Costs (Limit to 10% for those institutions requiring indirect funds. If not required enter "0%")					0%
				Indirect Costs	$0.00
TOTAL PROJECT BUDGET REQUEST					**$70,286.20**

Figure 16.2   Example of a quantitative research study budget

Federal research grants, unlike professional organizations, generally cover both direct and indirect costs, as well as base pay and fringe benefit rate, and a percentage of effort (% effort) for each member of the study team. Federal grants are often requested for larger, more complex studies and may include full-time personnel, high-tech equipment, laboratory studies, and other necessities. The bottom line is that the budgets are fairly similar; the scope of the project tends to define the size of the budget.

Finding Sources of Funding

There are many sources of research funding, as well as several different types of funding vehicles available to researchers who develop strong research studies. Thousands of private and public foundations and agencies support research. The funds, however, are not evenly distributed across disciplines, nor do they come without restrictions. A competitive proposal review is required by many funding sources, often resulting in the need for the submitter to make revisions to the prospective study proposal.

Look in Your Own Back Yard

When beginning to search for available research funding, don't forget to look within your own organization. Many larger institutions have a philanthropy department or development office, which serves as the fundraising arm of the institution. The philanthropy department develops relationships with community leaders in an effort to generate contributions from the community to fund special projects. Special projects may include building programs, research studies, or education programs, depending on the special interest of the donor. The professionals who work in this area are skilled in the process of finding and securing available funding. They may be an excellent resource for you as you search for research funding. In the absence of such a department, some organizations may have "special funds" that contain donated monies that have been designated for research, education, nursing excellence, or development. If your institution has a philanthropy department, or just a "special fund," be sure to check within your institution before seeking funding from exterior sources. Many institutions have fundraising policies and procedures that provide guidance for the researcher.

The researcher's previous performance, particularly as it relates to research and publication, weighs heavily among factors considered in awarding grants regardless of the funding source. One strategy for developing your track record so as to eventually receive a large grant award is to acquire two or three small ($2,000 to $5,000) research grants, conduct the studies, and publish study results. This strategy works well if you have a specific area of research interest and plan to build a program of research. A program of research is when one study builds upon the next, developing a body of knowledge on one topic rather than several studies conducted on an assortment of unrelated topics. This not only demonstrates to large research grant funders that you have the ability to successfully complete a study project, but that your work has already been critically reviewed and your ideas are worthy of major funding.

Federal Funding

The federal government is the largest source of research funding in the United States; the National Institutes of Health (NIH) and the Agency for Healthcare Research and Quality (AHRQ) are the leading agencies for health care research. Competitive proposal review is an integral part of the grant-making process. Funding may be received in the form of grants or contracts. Grants are "an award of funds without a fully defined set of terms and conditions for use, whereas a contract is a work order from the grantor in which procedures, costs, and funding period have been established in explicit terms" (Locke et al., 2000).

A researcher may learn of funding opportunities by one of several mechanisms. Regular grant programs are announced through Parent Announcements, and special opportunities are announced through Program Announcements, Requests for Applications (RFAs) for grants, and Requests for Proposals (RFPs) for contracts. Each mechanism provides information about a different type of funding. The Grants.gov website (http://grants.gov) provides a wealth of information about eligibility requirements, restrictions, grant details, and downloadable application forms. There are a number of different types of grants available from the National Institutes of Health (NIH) for which nurses may apply. Among the most common are the Research Project Grants (RO1), AREA Grants (R15), Small Grants (R03), or Exploratory/Developmental Grants (R21). Researchers complete and submit grant applications online. Each type of award has its own specific form to be completed and is evaluated by its own unique process. Such government-funded grants are highly competitive and are oftentimes awarded to researchers who have a proven track record of success, which can be very disappointing for novice researchers.

> **Q:** *I am looking for a grant in the amount of $2,500 to fund my first research study proposal. Should I apply for a National Institutes of Health grant?*

A: No, we would not recommend that you apply for a federal grant for your first research study. You are more likely to be successful if you apply for a small grant award through your institution, a professional nursing organization, or a non-nursing health organization.

Fewer than 25% of first-time applicants to NIH grants are successful (Locke et al., 2000). In addition, federal funding carries with it myriad monitoring and documentation requirements, many of which can be daunting to a novice researcher or to a researcher who does not have the support staff to ensure compliance with government regulations and auditing requirements. Many less-experienced researchers prefer to avoid government funding in order to not have to deal with the associated "red tape" and requirements, as well as to have a higher chance for success. For this reason, this chapter's focus is on nonfederal grant funding.

Nonfederal Funding

Nonfederal organizations provide promising opportunities for inexperienced researchers to fund research projects. Professional organizations, health organizations, and philanthropic foundations are excellent sources of research funding. Don't be surprised if membership in the organization is a requirement to applying for research funding from many professional nursing organizations.

Sigma Theta Tau International (STTI), the Honor Society of Nursing, offers an array of nursing research funding opportunities. It offers several different grants in which STTI partners with other professional nursing organizations, such as the Emergency Nurses Association Foundation and the Hospice and Palliative Nurses Foundation, to award research funding for qualifying nurse researchers. Awards range in size from $5,000 to $50,000 (www.nursingsociety.org/RESEARCH). In addition, many local STTI chapters award small grants of $1,000 to $4,000 to fund the research of chapter members. Professional nursing organizations are a rich source of research funding. Consider seeking funding from organizations like the national and local chapters of the American Organization of Nurse Executives, the American Association of Critical Care Nurses, the Oncology Nursing Society, and regional research societies (i.e. Western Institute of Nursing, Southern Nursing Research Society, etc.). Health organizations are also a strong source of research funding.

Nursing research is also promoted and supported by many non-nursing health organizations. Numerous well-known organizations—such as the American Diabetes Association, the American Heart Association, the Susan B. Komen Foundation, the American Hospital Association, and the American Cancer Association—establish research priorities and award funding to researchers whose study proposal addresses the organization's priorities. Information regarding research priorities and funding availability of health organizations, as well as philanthropic foundations, are usually available on the organization website, in their annual report, or through office personnel and board members of the local chapter.

Take Advantage of Google

Similarly, you can use the Google search engine on the Internet to identify such health organizations and foundations and then proceed to a website where you can find more information about their philanthropic priorities and programs, as well as names and contact information of agency personnel to contact regarding research priorities and deadlines.

After you have navigated the foundation's website, pay special attention to the foundation's charter, which establishes the organization's mission and designates their funding constraints. If the interests of the foundation align with your area of research, look for the foundation's funding priorities and a list of recent projects funded. Don't hesitate to contact the foundation for more information and for a grant application packet.

Adapting Your Proposal to Address the Funder's Priorities

When you have selected the funding agency that is best matched to you and your research project, it is time to adapt your research proposal to a grant proposal. Keeping in mind the funding agency's research priorities, grant requirements, and your specific needs, you should revise sections of the study proposal to align closely with the funding agency. We are not suggesting that you change the fundamental aim of the study or the chosen research methodology, but you should highlight the ways that your study aligns with the funding agency's research priorities. One way to do this is explained in the following example.

Let's say that you are looking for funding to support an education project in which you are teaching geriatric best practices to direct care staff nurses using a mixed methods approach. Two 8-hour workshops will be used to supply geriatric content, and you will teach evidence-based practice (EBP) project development skills in six monthly 8-hour days spread over a 6-month period of time. Participants will not only gain knowledge of geriatric best practices, but they will also learn to plan, develop and implement an evidence-based practice project. How can you change the focus of the proposal to align with the funding agency?

- When writing the grant proposal, if the funding agency is interested in funding geriatric projects you would highlight the use of geriatric best nursing practices in the proposal.

- If the grant agency is interested in funding innovative education projects, you would focus on the education methodologies employed in the project.

- You would highlight the growth and professional development of the staff nurse participants as they learn research and project development and management skills, if the funding agency prioritizes projects on nurse engagement and retention.

- By highlighting the EBP project development over the 6-month time span, the project aligns well with funders who prioritize translating research into practice.

By simply "putting on a different pair of glasses," you change the focus of the proposal to demonstrate to funders how the project "fits" with their research priorities. You are, in essence, "selling" them on the idea that your proposal is a great match for their organization.

Submitting a Grant Application

It is not uncommon for funding agencies to require the use of a specific proposal format. Be sure that you read the entire application packet before beginning the application, and follow the submission guidelines carefully. Guidelines may include items like required font type and size, spacing, type of paper, or method of handling tables and pictures. By following the regulations and meeting the deadlines, you may assume that your proposal will be reviewed. However, if you do not adhere to the regulations, chances are that your proposal may not be read, despite the quality of the project.

Foundation personnel can be particularly helpful in alerting you to deadlines, application procedures, and areas of particular interest to the foundation, as well as in describing the grant application review process and how final decisions are determined.

After the proposal submission process is complete, the review process gets underway. The proposal will be reviewed for scientific/technical merit, for alignment with the foundation's priorities, and by the perception of your ability to carry out the research study. In some organizations the review is conducted by a special committee of the board; in other organizations the review may be handled by outside experts. The grantor's decision is usually communicated to the applicant in a written email or letter.

When you've received the decision, be sure to respond to the grantor. If you were awarded the grant be sure to thank them. If the proposal was not funded be sure to request feedback from the review committee or the foundation personnel. Feedback is important for two reasons: It provides an opportunity for you to learn how to improve your proposal; and it may provide valuable information in case you decide to submit a proposal to the same foundation in the future.

Be sure to carefully consider the feedback that you've been given, and don't be afraid to incorporate it into your next proposal. Rejection does not necessarily mean that you don't have a good study proposal. It has grown more difficult to obtain research funding due to the increase in nurses who have obtained advanced degrees and the explosion of the use of EBP. There are many additional reasons for rejecting a grant proposal: timing of the award, the size of award requested, type of study, inexperience of the research team, number of grantees in your geographic location, or any number of other reasons. Whatever you do, don't get discouraged! Try, try again!

Research Funding Sources and Resources

Successful grant-seekers are those who have strong research and grantsmanship skills, write solid proposals, and know where to look for funding. Here are some good sources for fully funded grants:

- **Agency for Healthcare Research and Quality (AHRQ)**: A wealth of information can be found on the AHRQ Funding Opportunities website. It contains research policies, funding priorities, online submission forms, and training materials for grant submission, as well as announcements of new RFPs. Website: http://www.ahrq.gov/fund/

- **American Association of Critical Care Nurses (AACN):** Supports members of their organization who conduct research that supports bedside nurses to provide excellent quality care and ensure the safety of critically ill patients and their families. Funds support research studies that drive change in high acuity and critical care nursing practice. Awards range from $10,000 to $50,000. Website: http://www.aacn.org/WD/practice/content/grant-all.content?menu=Practice

- **American Nurses Association (ANA):** The ANA has a robust webpage of research grant opportunities. Whereas some are appropriate for novice researchers, others are intended for large-scale community health services research. Included in the list of "Other Prominent Funders for Consideration" are the Bill and Melinda Gates Foundation, the W. K. Kellogg Foundation, the Ford Foundation, and the Avon Foundation. Website: http://nursingworld.org/research-toolkit/Research-Funding

- **American Nurses Association, State and District Chapters:** In addition to the funding opportunities available from the national association, the state and district chapters offer smaller research awards. Be sure to check the website for further details.

- **Commerce Business Daily:** This website, which publishes a summary of federal RFPs, provides contract details for specific studies being requested by the government. Although it is not likely that an inexperienced researcher would be awarded such a contract, it is important that you know that the funding source exists. Website: http://cbdnet.gpo.gov

- **Federal Government:** This website is a central storehouse for information on more than 1,000 grant programs and provides access to approximately $500 billion in annual awards. Many categories of organizations are eligible to apply for government grants: government, education, public housing organizations, small businesses, and nonprofit and for-profit organizations. Individuals may also apply for a government grant. An individual submits a grant on their own behalf, and not on behalf of a company, organization, institution, or government. Individuals sign the grant application and its associated certifications and assurances that are necessary to fulfill the requirements of the application process. So, if you register as an individual, you are only able to apply to grant opportunities that are open to individuals. An individual cannot submit a grant application to a grant opportunity that is open only to organizations. Go to http://www.grants.gov/assets/GrantsGov_Applicant_UserGuide_R12.1.0_V2.1.pdf for the Applicant User Guide. Website: http://www.grants.gov

- **Foundation Center:** This website provides a wealth of information about philanthropic foundations that fund research. It also holds seminars and training on grant writing and funding at various locations throughout the United States Website: http://www.fdncenter.org/findfunders/

The Foundation Directory Online (http://fconline.foundationcenter.org/) is a comprehensive, fee-based online resource for identifying funding opportunities that can be found on the Foundation Center website. The directory contains the names, purpose, activities, and contact information for philanthropic foundations that fund research.

- **Health Services Research Information Central:** The website of the National Information Center on Health Services Research and Health Care Technology (NICHSR) serves the information needs of the health services research community. The website provides information about grants, fellowships and funding opportunities for federal, foundation, and other funding sources. Website: http://www.nlm.nih.gov/hsrinfo/grantsites.html#322FundingOpportunities

- **National Institute of Nursing Research (NINR):** This federal program is under the umbrella of NIH and the division of Health and Human Services. In addition to funding opportunities, the website announces requests for proposals and maintains lists of funded research programs. This provides you with the opportunity to explore the types of research funded and the monetary amount of each award. Website: https://www.ninr.nih.gov/researchandfunding

- **Sigma Theta Tau International (STTI):** The Honor Society of Nursing provides grant opportunities in addition to cosponsored grants with other professional organizations. There are numerous grant vehicles for which a researcher might apply. The newest grant award is the Sigma Theta Tau International Global Nursing Research Grant and is intended to encourage nurses to focus on responding to health disparities globally. Funding is awarded on the basis of the quality of the proposed research study, the applicant's research budget, and the applicant's potential as a nurse scientist. Funding is awarded up to a maximum of $12,000. Website: http://www.nursingsociety.org/Research/Grants/Pages/Grantsbydate.aspx

Cosponsored grants include the following:

- **Southern Nursing Research Society (SNRS) Research Grant:** The purpose of the grant is to encourage qualified nurses to contribute to the science of nursing. They consider proposals for pilot studies as well as development research studies. Application deadline is April 1st. Website: http://www.snrs.org/i4a/pages/index.cfm?pageid=3282

- **Emergency Nurses Association Foundation (ENAF) Grant:** This grant encourages nursing research that will benefit the practice of emergency nursing. Studies that align with the ENA/ENA Foundation Research initiatives are given priority. Application deadline is March 1st. Website: http://www.internationalscholarships.com/389/Emergency-Nursing-Foundation-Grant

- **Rehabilitation Nursing Foundation Grant:** Funds research proposals that address the clinical practice, educational, or administrative dimensions of rehabilitation nursing. Requires that the PI hold a master's degree. Application deadline is March 1st. Website: http://www.rehabnurse.org/research/content/RNF-Research-Grants.html

- **Association of Nurses in AIDS Care (ANAC) Grant:** This grant is intended to encourage clinically oriented HIV/AIDS research and to increase the number of nursing research studies that focus on HIV prevention, symptom management, promotion of self-care, and adherence. Application deadline is April 1st. Website: http://www.nursingsociety.org/Research/Grants/Pages/anac_grant.aspx

- **Association of periOperative Registered Nurses (AORN) Grant:** The purpose of this grant is to encourage the conduct of research related to nursing practice in the perioperative setting and to build the science of perioperative nursing. Priority is given to research studies that relate to the AORN research priorities. Application deadline is April 1st. Website: http://www.nursingsociety.org/Research/Grants/Pages/grant_aorn.aspx

- **Hospice and Palliative Nurses Foundation End of Life Nursing Care Research (HPNF) Grant:** This grant is intended to encourage qualified nurses to conduct research that contributes to the advancement of nursing care. Funding is available for both pilot studies and developmental research. The application deadline is April 1st. Website: http://www.hpnf.org/DisplayPage.aspx?Title=Research%20Grants

- **American Nurses' Foundation (ANF) Grant:** The purpose of this grant is to support the studies of beginning nurse researchers or that of experienced nurse researchers who are entering a new field of study. Awards are available in many areas of nursing; among them are women's health, gerontology, community and family intervention, healthy patient outcomes, health care policy, and critical care. Application deadline is May 1st. Website: http://www.anfonline.org/MainCategory/NursingResearchGrant.aspx

Try It Now!

Develop a budget to display the cost of conducting this nursing research study:

A researcher has designed a randomized control study in which study participants are asked to complete a demographic questionnaire and answer the Spielberger's State-Trait Anxiety Inventory (STAI) questionnaire. The download for a total of 250 copies of the STAI will cost $200, and it will require about three reams of paper at $5.00 per ream on which to print two copies of the STAI for each participant. The State-Trait Anxiety Inventory for Adults Manual, which is required for scoring the questionnaires, costs $40.00. A music library consisting of 16 MP3 players, which have been preloaded with different music selections, will be available; they cost $30.00 each, plus tax, for a total of $520.80. Headphones for the MP3 players must also be purchased; a total of 16 sets at $10 each, plus tax, totals $173.20. Disposable earphone covers cost $17 for a package of 100; 300 ear covers plus tax totals $55.34. The kinds of music that will be offered are nonlyrical religious, classical, jazz, and natural sounds; the cost of the music downloads is $24.45. Participants will be asked to choose from the music collection to select the preferred music genre. Participants in the control group will receive the standard of care based upon the unit's routine care delivery process. Participants who belong to the first group will be assigned the 30-minute music intervention, the second group the 15-minute intervention, and the third group as the control group will receive no music. Immediately following the music intervention, the participants will be asked to complete the STAI for the second time. The control group will be asked to complete the STAI after resting for 30 minutes. The research team will consist of four select staff nurses in the Day Surgery Unit who will enroll and consent study participants. Each research team member will receive a $50 gift card as an incentive to assist the PI with the study.

References

Agency for Healthcare Research and Quality (AHRQ). Retrieved from http://www.ahrq.gov/fund/

American Association of Critical Care Nurses (AACN). Retrieved from http://www.aacn.org/WD/practice/content/grant-all.content?menu=Practice

Grami, P., & Smith, C. D. (Unpublished). Establishing the proportion of patients with acute delirium and evaluating the feasibility and effectiveness of a delirium.

Grants.gov. Retrieved from www.grants.gov

Locke, L. F., Spirduso, W. W., & Silverman, S. J. (2000). *Proposals that work: A guide for planning dissertations and grant proposals.* Thousand Oaks, CA: Sage Publications.

McClurkin, S. (Unpublished). An exploration of the duration of self-selected music in reducing preoperative anxiety.

Sigma Theta Tau International Honor Society of Nursing. Retrieved from www.nursingsociety.org/RESEARCH

"If I walk my dog in the park, this is considered a public act. Is that act similar to posting a Facebook photo when my privacy setting is selected as 'To All'? In either case, am I a potential research subject without knowing it?"

–Jane Bliss-Holtz

17

Research, the Internet, and Social Media: Powerful Resource or Perilous Endeavor?

Jane Bliss-Holtz

WHAT YOU'LL LEARN IN THIS CHAPTER

- Recruiting research subjects using social media is a worthwhile approach, but there are issues related to using social media for recruitment.

- Web-based survey applications, which are more commonly used in research, have several advantages over paper-and-pencil data collection.

- The use of paradata may allow for construction of a more reliable survey instrument.

Use of the Internet and related social media to deliver patient education, to monitor patient adherence to health care regimes, and as an alternative delivery method of prelicensure and professional education has increased within the last 20 years. However, as use of the Internet as a data source and as a medium for data collection also has begun to increase, it has only been within recent years that issues related to data ownership, data security, and assurance (or the lack thereof) of confidentiality have been raised. Although the same basic quantitative research designs that have been described throughout this book have been used in Internet and social media research, how data are captured and stored can be quite different. Additionally, in the case of qualitative research, the use of available Facebook pages, web pages, Twitter "tweets," YouTube videos, and instant messages as data sources brings into focus the complexity of these issues. Although the purpose of this chapter is to describe the use of the Internet and selected social media for research purposes, as well as to identify some of the related challenges, it must be realized that the issues are as fluid as the medium in which they occur.

The Definition of Social Media

Social media is a mode of communication that is Internet-based and enables participants to interact with the medium and/or users of the medium. Social media encompasses activities such as (Parrish & Carbary, 2011):

- Social networking (examples include Facebook and Twitter)

- Photograph and video sharing (examples include YouTube and Shutterfly)

- Online journaling (blogs)

- Audiocasting (podcasts)

- Audiovisual media (webcasting)

Within the realm of social media also exist Internet-based applications that have been increasingly used in research, including SurveyMonkey, which has incorporated Zoomerang; Polldaddy; and Poll Everywhere. These web-based applications include basic (and free) options that allow for creating, administering, and analyzing a limited number of survey responses. (These applications are discussed later in this chapter in the section "Commercial Web-based Survey Applications.")

Q: *I am back in school for my master's degree and need to do a capstone project. I'm interested in workplace violence as a topic and plan to use one of the free web-based survey tools to send a survey to the nurses who work with me in our emergency department (ED) about the types and frequency of workplace violence that they encounter. Because the survey is on the Internet and I won't be distributing the survey at work, do I need to go to my hospital's Institutional Review Board (IRB)? I'm just going to ask the nurses if they are interested and send them the link via email if they are.*

A: For numerous reasons, the answer is, "Yes, you need IRB approval." Even though the actual survey will be distributed on the Internet and not at work, you will be recruiting your subjects from your hospital's ED; therefore you need to have the project reviewed by the IRB. In addition, the IRB will be assessing the items on the survey because, depending on what questions are being asked, this topic is potentially sensitive in nature and may need a full review to assure that privacy and confidentiality of the subjects are being fully protected. (Also see Chapter 14 in the book.) They also may want information about the security of the survey site being used, so choose your site carefully. You might want to consider making your first stop your hospital's nursing research committee. They could advise you on IRB procedure, as well as tell you who else you might need to notify, such as the chief nurse executive and the appropriate department heads.

Facebook as an Example of Social Media and Its Research Uses

Facebook, which started as a social network exclusively for Harvard University students, has evolved into a social networking site that "went public" in an initial public offering (IPO) on February 1, 2012. As of July 20, 2013 Facebook reported having more than 1.5 billion active users, with almost 700 million daily active users reported by the end of June 2013 (Facebook Newsroom, 2013).

Although Facebook started as a social network, businesses have found Facebook an important route to potential customers, as marketers can select the location, gender, age, likes and interests, relationship status, workplace, and education of their target audience. Because of this ability to use the information that Facebook collects to selectively target audiences, investigators have increasingly used Facebook and similar social media to recruit research subjects (Fenner et al., 2012). Through use of the Internet, investigators have access to large numbers of individuals who can be contacted in a cost-effective way (Ramo, Hall, & Prochaska, 2010). Additionally, through use of Facebook user groups, researchers can locate and approach subjects who may otherwise be hard to reach (Greeley et al., 2011; Levine et al., 2011).

Research Subject Recruitment

An example of the use of social media in recruiting subjects is that of Balfe, Doyle, and Conroy (2012), who described their experience with using Facebook to recruit young adults (aged 23 to 30 years) with type 1 diabetes for participation in a qualitative study exploring their thoughts about diabetes health care services in Ireland. The recruiting results, discussed next, exemplify some of the methodological issues related to "recruiting on the 'Net.'"

During the short study time frame of 12 months, the investigators were able to gain ethics approval for recruitment from only one hospital. As the target number of subjects to recruit and interview was 40, and recruitment from only one hospital would not allow for results that would be transferable to a nationwide population, the investigators decided to place a recruitment message on the Diabetes Ireland Facebook (DIF) page, which, at the time, had approximately 1,500 members. They also placed a message on the page of a support group of young Irish adults, which had approximately 220 members. Four recruitment messages were placed 2 to 3 weeks apart on each site. In addition, the investigators were able to search the membership list of the young Irish adult support group and sent 50 members a private Facebook invitation and a follow-up message one week later.

A total of 26 subjects were recruited from DIF recruitment, with an additional two participants added via *snowball recruiting* (referral) from DIF members. None were recruited from the young Irish adult support group, despite the personalized invitations. Within the same time period, only seven participants were recruited from the hospital setting. Thus, of 35 subjects recruited, only 20% were recruited from the hospital and 80% were recruited (through various strategies) from the Facebook social media site. The investigators commented that recruitment through social media was "lower and slower" than hoped, given the large number of individuals that the media had reached (Balfe et al., 2012), however the rate was similar to that shown in earlier literature (Fenner et al., 2012; Levine et al., 2011; Tan, 2010).

An unexpected issue was that, although overrecruiting from only one hospital was avoided, the final sample was rather homogeneous, which was the threat to the ability to transfer the findings to the more general population of diabetics that the investigators originally sought to avoid by turning to Facebook recruitment (Balfe et al., 2012). Of those recruited, 26 (74%) were women and 30 (86%) were educated at least with a bachelor's degree. Those recruited from Facebook also had fairly good control of their diabetes.

This issue of overrepresentation of more affluent and educated social media users also has been reported by Zickuhr and Smith (2012) in a recent Pew Research Center report and will continue to be an issue when subjects are recruited through social media. One strategy that would assist in overcoming the challenge of a skewed sample is the use of quota sampling, in which characteristics that might have an influence on the study results are identified, the percentage of their presence in the total population is determined, and then a sample is recruited that mimics this percentage.

For example, if investigators are concerned that socioeconomic status might influence study results, and they find that the general population consists of 20% upper, 60% middle, and 20% lower socioeconomic status, then they would need to recruit a sample comprised of 20% upper, 60% middle, and 20% lower socioeconomic status. Im & Chee (2011) reported that quota sampling was considered; however, several practical issues in the use of quota sampling negated its use, including difficulty in reaching lower socioeconomic groups; difficulty in authenticating sensitive demographic information, such as incongruence between answers to screening questions and final survey responses; and the annoyance of volunteers when they are not chosen.

Another unexpected finding by Balfe and associates (2012) was that the dropout rate was much lower in the Facebook participants when compared to those recruited from the hospital setting. It was suggested that this may have occurred because Facebook participants felt no threat to their health care, thus they had no feeling of coercion upon originally agreeing to participate.

Social Media as Data

Social media not only has been used as a vehicle for research subject recruitment, but as a data source as well. An example of this is found in a research report by Egan and Moreno (2011), who used a Facebook search to identify 300 public Facebook profiles of undergraduate freshmen at a large Midwestern state university. A subsequent content analysis was performed of Facebook content to identify references to stress, concerns about weight, depression, and alcohol use. During the study, demographic data, including age, sex, and dates of first and most recent Facebook activity, were collected from the self-reported personal information pages (Walls) of Facebook profiles. Data analysis included content coding of all publicly available personal information, which included group affiliations, status updates, "bumper stickers," and any photographs of the profile owner. Content coding was performed using a code book that defined terms that were considered references to stress, weight concerns, depressive symptoms, and alcohol use. The authors suggested that by using this venue, students at risk for stress-related conditions could be identified and that targeted information about stress-relief resources could be delivered to them.

Using the Internet as a Medium for Data Collection

The most widely used commercial Internet survey applications include SurveyMonkey (http://www.surveymonkey.com), Polldaddy (http://www.polldaddy.com), and Poll Everywhere (http://www.polleverywhere.com). Depending on the plan chosen, these applications allow investigators to:

- Develop surveys

- Collect responses through a dedicated website (the survey link can be placed in emails, in social media, or on a dedicated website) or directly in Facebook, Twitter, or on an iPad

- Download data for analysis

Although most investigators opt for one of several data plans, these web-based applications include basic options that allow for creation, administration, and analysis of a limited number of survey responses for no fee, which is a reason you may want to use it in a small study with a limited budget. See Table 17.1 for a comparison of these applications.

Table 17.1   Comparison of Free User Option for Surveys: SurveyMonkey, Polldaddy, and Poll Everywhere

Feature	SurveyMonkey	Polldaddy	Poll Everywhere
Users	1 user	1 user	1 user
Number of Questions	10 questions	10 questions	Not stated in website
Number of Responders	100 respondents/ survey	200/month	40 respondents/ survey
Data Analysis/Reports	Limited reports available	Reports available for polls, surveys, and quizzes	Limited to no automatic reports
Advertising	"Powered by SuveryMonkey" on footer of survey	Content will contain Polldaddy links	Not stated in website
Additional Information	Security not enhanced Does not allow data export	Does not allow data export	Does not allow data export; security at same level for all users

Web-based surveys have several advantages over paper-and-pencil data collection, including the following:

- Skip patterns (these allow for automatic skipping over irrelevant questions such as if nurses answer that they have no certification, the next question that asks which certification has been attained is skipped)

- Prohibition of out-of-range responses through use of fixed choice items (drop-down menus)

- Safeguards against missing or skipping items by not allowing the user to continue until all questions on a screen are completed.

Additionally, potential errors in data entry are avoided, as data are directly entered and stored in a database (Sowan & Jenkins, 2010).

Culley (2011) and Holloway (2012) described a creative use of online survey tools. Both authors used online survey tools to conduct a Delphi (or *e-Delphi*) survey, which is an iterative process through which expert panel consensus is (hopefully) reached. When an expert panel is identified and members have agreed to participate, initial statements derived from literature and other key documents and stakeholder interviews are rated or ranked, and responses are then compiled. These compiled responses are shared in a second round with the panel participants, who are asked to rate or rank statements a second time. When a pre-set level of agreement is reached, consensus is considered to have been obtained. Benefits of using an online tool in Delphi surveys included data analysis support; cost-effectiveness, especially when multiple rounds of surveys are conducted; geographic flexibility; and use of email for initial recruitment contact (Holloway 2012).

Generation of Paradata From Web-Administered Measures

Placing data collection tools online gives investigators the ability not only to gather data related to the research question, but also to collect information related to how users respond to the tool. This becomes important when a survey is created, as paradata can indicate how user-friendly the survey is, which increases the chances of capturing a better return rate, something that is always a challenge when launching a survey. As usability of an instrument contributes to the ability to assess its reliability and validity, this information is valuable to researchers.

Coined by Couper (2000), the term *paradata* is used to refer to this "byproduct" data that can be used to evaluate the usability of web-administered tools. Server-side paradata that can be collected includes:

- The total number of visits to the instrument

- The time spent by each respondent

- The Internet protocol (IP) addresses and respondent identifiers, if used, for site access

- The browser and operating system version used

Client-side paradata includes information about the behavior patterns of respondents and can include:

- Data related to number of response changes for each item

- The length of time spent on each item

- The sequence of item response (where flexibility is given)

- How skip patterns were followed (Sowan & Jenkins, 2010)

Analysis of both types of paradata enables investigators to make refinements in response formats, question sequence and skip patterns, and general layout of the instrument, thus improving the reliability and validity of the measurement.

Online Synchronous Focus Groups

You can use real-time synchronous online focus groups to mimic the group interaction of face-to-face focus groups without the risk of exposure to other participants or to the investigator. Group interaction is in real-time; when one person types a question or a response to a question, the text immediately pops up on the computer screen, enabling other group members to read and respond to it.

Using proprietary software such as InterQue (http://crusader-services. com/froups.shtml), investigators can send to participants passwords that are generated directly by the software program, assuring participant anonymity. Additionally, InterQue has the option of providing secure, randomly selected anonymous entry into the chat room and has a "double-sided" screen, assuring that participants are not identified through use of the program.

Lessening the threat to anonymity can lead to more willingness to volunteer for group participation and to easier disclosure of sensitive information (Stover, 2012). Another benefit to using such software is that transcripts are available almost immediately for download into plain ASCII text or spreadsheet-ready tab separated values (TSV) files, thus reducing the possibility of transcription error. The software might also include the ability to time-stamp the transcripts and to sort them by participant.

Issues in the Use of Social Media and the Internet in Research

With the increase in research that uses existing social media as data or to recruit subjects and/or collect data from subjects, issues related to these uses have surfaced. For example, debate continues on whether social media data are located in a true "public setting" and, therefore, whether an IRB review is necessary. Use of paradata has its own collection-related issues, including users not knowing that their IP addresses, usernames, and passwords might be collected as data. Finally, as "hacker attacks" become more and more sophisticated, data storage security "in the cloud" has become a deeper concern. The following sections explore these issues in more depth.

Using Social Media and Internet Content as Data

As previously discussed, Egan and Moreno (2011) described use of a Facebook search to identify the public Facebook profiles of undergraduate freshmen at a large Midwestern state university and subsequent use of their Facebook pages as data to analyze the frequency of stress references. Because of the growing concern for privacy, the default settings on Facebook have been revised since the time that the study data were collected in 2009. Among other changes, Facebook profiles that are set as fully private by their profile owners no longer appear in Facebook searches for random profiles (Egan & Moreno, 2011).

The ethical considerations of using social media as data are considerable. Some investigators would argue that use of this media is similar to performing observations in a public setting. Additionally, users of social media choose to set levels of accessibility through privacy settings. Using this line of thinking, then, if information is made available "to all," then it was done by the act of the user. Continuing this line of thinking, research conducted using this data might be considered exempt by an IRB (Moreno, Fost, & Christakis, 2008). However, when Internet and social media content are used as data, issues of confidentiality need to be considered in reporting the findings (see Chapter 14 for a full discussion of these concepts).

Although the content is public, research findings should not reveal any linkages between personal identifiers and potentially damaging information, as this would constitute secondary disclosure of information (Moreno et al., 2011).

> **Q:** *I am planning a qualitative study that will involve searching health care websites and analyzing their content related to consumer advice about commonly occurring infections and use of specific antibiotics. Do I need to go to my IRB for review?*

> **A:** It seems as though your research would fall under the category of *exempt* review. This is defined as research that involves the collection or study of existing data or documents that are publicly available (and Internet webpages certainly fit that qualification). That being said, you cannot simply decide that your study is exempt—the proposal still needs to be submitted to your institution's IRB, as that body is the only one that can make that determination.

Another issue is that of obtaining a "representative sample" from social media. In this, investigators have to do their homework as far as being aware of what current social media demographics might be. For example, if the target population for a study is adolescents and young adults, then knowing that 65% of Internet users between 12 and 17 years use social media would be useful in gauging the possible demographics of a sample recruited from social media (Zickuhr & Smith, 2012). Conversely, target populations of adults aged older than 45 years recruited from social media may not be representative, as less than 23% of adults over the age of 45 years use social media (Zickuhr & Smith, 2012).

Collection and Use of Paradata

Ethical issues related to the use of paradata is an area that is still being explored, especially when paradata are collected without the knowledge of participants. Although not generally known by users, server-side paradata are automatically compiled in educational software used in online education, as well as in commercial web-based measurement applications (Sowan & Jenkins, 2010). Keep in mind that this data may include IP addresses, which can be used to identify users' "home" computers (although not necessarily the individual user), as well as other respondent information such as usernames and/or passwords that were used to access the site; thus, paradata cannot be considered anonymous information.

Prudent investigators who plan on collecting and using paradata should consult with their IRBs to discuss protection of the rights of human research subjects. Reporting of paradata findings follow the same ethical considerations as that of any research—that no individual respondent identifiers are linked to the paradata in the report. Similarly, the standards for data security and access of paradata are the same as they are for all research data.

Data Security and Access

Advances in wireless connectivity, the increased ability to encrypt data transfer, and increasingly sophisticated security systems have allowed for data storage in a centralized location while still allowing access to the data from multiple sites (Musick et al., 2011). As with any research data, access to electronic databases should be restricted to that of the research team, with security of the data assured by such measures as secure socket layer (SSL) data encryption upon transfer, multiple levels of permission, data redundancy, and detailed data backup and disaster recovery plans.

It is becoming more common for IRBs to require documentation of secure data transmission for multisite research studies. It also is not unusual for investigators planning multisite research to identify the level of access that all members of the research team will have to the data. For example, a core team member may have access to all areas of a database, whereas a statistician may only have access to data that is void of personal identifiers, such as subject identification number or date of birth. In addition, there may be additional security measures (such as security questions or secondary passwords) for access by research team members from remote locations.

Questions about data security have also arisen related to commercial web-based survey applications, as data stored by these sites needs to be secure and accessible only to the research team. Each survey application being considered should be evaluated for its security statements, which should be easy to locate. For example, at http://www.surveymonkey.com/mp/policy/security, you can find the security statement for SurveyMonkey. At minimum, when evaluating a security statement made by a commercial web-based data collection and storage site, the information that you should look for in the statement is presented in Table 17.2.

Table 17.2   Security Statement Topics That Should Be Evaluated in Commercial Web-Based Data Collection and Storage Sites

Security Topic	Areas Included
User Security	Use of user-generated usernames and passwords
	Creation of session cookies without usernames/passwords
	Use of SSL technology for data encryption and credit transactions
Physical Security	Service Organization Control (SOC) audits are performed in the facility
	Data center is physically secured by pass cards or biometrics
	Digital and environmental surveillance and control (humidity, smoke, heat) is used
	Servers are locked
	Country of server location is considered stable
Availability of Data	Servers have redundant internal and external power sources
	Multiple routing of Internet connections (Tier I Internet access provision)
	Failover time (time between failure of a primary server and full initiation of a back-up system) is acceptable to the project
	System uptime (e.g., whether the server is running) is continuously monitored
Network Security	Firewalls are used to restrict port access
	Intrusion detection systems are in place that monitor for outside intruders
	Network security audits are performed routinely (on a weekly basis is considered standard)
	Viral and malware scans are performed daily
Storage Security	Encrypted data backups occur on a regular basis both internally and externally in intervals acceptable to the project
	Level of RAID (Redundant Array of Independent Disks) used (RAID 0 means that there is no data redundancy; RAID 10 indicates excellent "mission critical" data redundancy; Natarajan, 2010).
Software Security	Latest patches are applied to all operating systems as they are made available

Try It Now!

Sign up for a free subscription to one of the commercial web-based survey applications. After reviewing the tutorial, think of five demographic areas (e.g., age, gender, nursing specialty, type of certification, etc.) about which you might want to collect data, and decide which features available in the survey would best be used to collect data on each one. Design your questions and see how they "work." If you're brave, send your survey out to several colleagues and see how the application reports the results.

References

Balfe, M., Doyle, F., & Conroy, R. (2012). Using Facebook to recruit young adults for qualitative research projects: How difficult is it? *CIN: Computers, Informatics, Nursing, 30*(11), 511–515.

Couper, M. (2000). Usability evaluation of computer assisted research instruments. *Social Science Computer Review, 18*(4), 384–396.

Crusader Services. Retrieved from http://crusader-services.com/froups.shtml

Culley, J. M. (2011). Use of a computer-mediated Delphi process to validate a mass casualty conceptual model. *CIN: Computers, Informatics, Nursing, 29*(5), 272–279.

Egan, K. G., & Moreno, M. A. (2011). Prevalence of stress references on college freshmen Facebook profiles. *CIN: Computers, Informatics, Nursing, 29*(10), 586–592.

Facebook Newsroom (2013). Retrieved from http://newsroom.fb.com/Key-Facts

Fenner, Y., Garland, S. M., Moore, E. E., Jayasinghe, Y., Fletcher, A., Tabrizi, S. N., & Wark, J. D. (2012). Web-based recruiting for health research using a social networking site: An exploratory study. *Journal of Medical Internet Research,14*(1), e20. Retrieved from http://www.ncbi.nlm.nih.gov/pmc/articles/PMC3374531

Greeley, S. A., Naylor, R. N., Cook, L. S., Tucker S. E., Lipton, R. B., & Philipson, L. H. (2011). Creation of the web-based University of Chicago Monogenic Diabetes Registry: Using technology to facilitate longitudinal study of rare subtypes of diabetes. *Journal of Diabetes Science and Technology, 5*(4), 879–886. Retrieved from http://www.ncbi.nlm.nih.gov/pmc/articles/PMC3192593

Holloway, K. (2012). Doing the E-Delphi: Using online survey tools. *CIN: Computers, Informatics, Nursing, 30*(7), 347–350.

Im, E-O., & Chee, W. (2011). Quota sampling in Internet research. *CIN: Computers, Informatics, Nursing, 29*(7), 381–385.

Levine, D., Madsen, A., Wright, E., Barar, R. E., Santelli, J., & Bull, S. (2011). Formative research on MySpace: Online methods to engage hard-to-reach populations. *Journal of Health Communication, 16*(4), 448–454.

Moreno, M. A., Fost, M. C., & Christakis, D. A. (2008). Research ethics in the MySpace era. *Pediatrics, 121*(1), 157–161.

Musick, B. S., Robb, S. L., Burns, D. S., Stegenga, K., Van, M., McCorkle, K. J. & Haase, J. E. (2011). Development and use of a web-based data management system for a randomized clinical trial of adolescents and young adults. *CIN: Computers, Informatics, Nursing, 29*(6), 337–343.

Natarajan, R. (2010). RAID 0, RAID 1, RAID 5, RAID 10 explained with diagrams. *The Geek Stuff.* Retrieved from http://www.thegeekstuff.com/2010/08/raid-levels-tutorial

Parrish, M. E., & Carbary, J. C. (2011). Using social media in research: Regulatory and IRB considerations. Retrieved from http://www.quorumreview.com/social-media-research-regulatory-irb-considerations

Ramo, D., Hall, S., & Prochaska, J. (2010). Reaching young adult smokers through the Internet: Comparison of three recruitment mechanisms. *Nicotine & Tobacco Research, 12*(7), 768–775.

Sowan, A. K., & Jenkins, L. S. (2010). Paradata: A new data source from web-administered measures. *CIN: Computers, Informatics, Nursing, 28*(6), 333–342.

Stover, C. M. (2012). The use of online synchronous focus groups in a sample of lesbian, gay, and bisexual college students. *CIN: Computers, Informatics, Nursing, 30*(8), 395–399.

Tan, H. (2010). Recruitment of participants using Facebook. In H. Forgasz & S. Groves (Eds.), *Contemporary approaches to research in mathematics, science, health and environmental education: Conference and symposium proceedings* (5th ed.). Geelong, Victoria, Australia: Deakin University, Centre for Studies in Mathematics, Science and Environmental Education, 1–5.

Zickuhr, K., & Smith, A. (2012). *Digital differences.* Pew Research Center's Internet & American Life Project Report. Washington, DC: Pew Research Center. Retrieved from http://pewinternet.org/ Reports/2012/ Digital-differences.aspx

Glossary

abstract   A brief written synopsis of the research project. Abstracts include a description of the problem, methods, results, and conclusions of the project.

abstraction tool   Lists all the study variables, and the variables are listed in the order they are found in the medical record/dataset.

alpha   The significance level (usually 0.05) selected by the researcher; the probability of incorrectly rejecting the null hypothesis.

anonymity   Data cannot be linked in any way with the identity of the participant, even by the researcher.

ANOVA (Analysis of Variance)   Compares the differences between the groups (numerator) to the differences within the groups (denominator), which produces an F statistic with a corresponding p value.

assent   Affirmative agreement to participate in research; used in conjunction with proxy consent if a potential participant is determined to lack capacity to consent to the research project.

autonomy   An individual's self-determination and freedom to make judgments as to what will be done to their person.

Boolean operators   An operation used during an electronic search to combine two or more key concepts; usually AND, OR, and NOT.

Chi-Square test   A statistical test that looks for a difference or association in two or more independent samples when the outcome variable is at the nominal or ordinal level; produces χ^2 and corresponding probability, or p value.

clinical significance   A statistically significant difference that is also determined by the experts in the field to be clinically useful.

cluster sampling   Randomly selects a group/unit/facility and then assigns either all or a random selection of the chosen group as the sample.

code book   A system of words used to define variables that summarize your data.

coercion   In research, applying influence, intimidation, or force on a subject to participate in the study.

comparative study   A study design that compares variables or subjects.

confidentiality   Data may be separated from the subject's identifying information, but the researcher can still link the data to the individual subject.

content validity   Describes whether the instrument is accurately measuring the full domain (content) of a concept, characteristic, or trait.

construct validity   Describes the degree to which the instrument measures the construct or trait.

convenience sampling   A sample that nonrandomly selects the most convenient subjects for the study.

correlation coefficient   The strength of the correlation; ranges from –1 to +1.

correlational design   A study design that examines the association or relationship between or among variables.

criterion-related validity   Describes how the performance on a measure relates to the "gold standard."

Cronbach's alpha   A reliability estimate of internal consistency of an instrument.

cross-sectional design   A method used to measure subjects at one point in time.

data coding   The translation of data into labeled categories suitable for computer processing.

data saturation   The point during data collection and analysis when no new information is forthcoming from participants.

decision-making capacity   The ability to make a reasoned choice.

Delphi (e-Delphi) survey   An iterative process through which expert panel consensus is (hopefully) reached.

dependent variable   The outcome variable or final result.

descriptive statistics   Sample values that summarize the properties of the data set.

directional hypothesis A hypothesis that identifies a direction to "look for" in the data that is collected; also called *one-tailed hypothesis*.

dissemination The act of sharing the results of completed research or research in progress. Main avenues for dissemination include oral and poster presentations, as well as published manuscripts.

effect size A statistical expression of the strength of a relationship between the study variables.

ethnography A type of qualitative study that focuses on the behaviors or "ways of life" of people in a particular culture.

evidence-based practice (EBP) An approach to clinical decision-making that incorporates (a) a systematic search for, critical appraisal, and synthesis of the most relevant and best research (i.e., external evidence) to answer a burning clinical question; (b) one's own clinical expertise, which includes internal evidence generated from outcomes management or quality improvement projects, a thorough patient assessment, and evaluation and use of available resources necessary to achieve desired patient outcomes; and (c) patient values and preferences.

exclusion criteria A characteristic or set of characteristics that restricts the subject from being chosen from the sampling frame, promoting homogeneity (similarity).

experimental design A study design that seeks to establish a cause-and-effect relationship.

external validity The extent to which the study findings can be generalized from the study sample to a larger population.

extraneous/confounding variables Variables that may have an indirect effect on the dependent variable, but are not the independent variable.

field notes Notes written by a researcher after each interview that includes information such as observations about the participant, the setting, and/or interactions that occur during the interview.

frequency The numerical counts of a value or category of a measurement.

generalizability The extent to which sample findings can be applied to the population from which the sample was drawn.

grant In research, the funding secured to carry out the study.

grantsmanship   The use of a set of skills associated with developing a fundable proposal.

grounded theory   A type of qualitative study that focuses on a social process in which a theory is developed that is grounded in the descriptions of participants.

hypothesis   An observation or research idea that can be tested.

implementation science   Conducting research to determine which strategies are the most efficient to get an evidence-based intervention *sustainably* into practice.

inclusion criteria   A characteristic or set of population characteristics necessary for inclusion in the study.

independent variable   A variable measured or controlled by the experimenter; the variable the researcher believes may be related to the outcome.

inferential statistics   The process of drawing conclusions about a population based on the measurements obtained in a sample.

informed consent   A process by which a subject has agreed to participate in a research study. A signed informed consent document is evidence that the subject has participated in the process, including explanation of the study, and has agreed.

Institutional Review Board (IRB)   The approval committee that has organizational oversight for the protection of human subjects.

internal validity   The extent to which the independent variable, and not something else, effects the dependent variable.

internal consistency reliability   Describes a mechanism by which all of the items within an instrument capture the concept; also referred to as *homogeneity*.

inter-rater reliability   Ensures that the results of an instrument would provide equivalent results if performed by another person.

interval measurement   Level of measurement with equal distances between points on a scale and no meaningful zero.

Likert scale   A type of self-report measure in which a subject chooses a response indicating a degree of agreement or disagreement with a statement.

literature review   Orients the reader to what is known and not known about the topic of interest.

longitudinal design   A method used to measure subjects over time.

mean   The sum of the values divided by the total number of observations; also known as the *average*; the mean is the most commonly reported measure of central tendency.

measurement   In quantitative research, the process of assigning a numerical value to data.

measurement error   The difference between the real value and the value obtained.

measures of central tendency   Describes how the values of a variable cluster.

median   A measure of central tendency that lines up all the measured values in order from least to most; the median is the value in the middle.

McNemar's test   Similar to a Chi-square test, but accommodates the dependency of the samples; produces a McNemar's test statistic χ^2 and a corresponding p value.

minimal risk   The probability and magnitude of harm or discomfort anticipated in the research are not greater in and of themselves than those ordinarily encountered in daily life.

mode   A measure of central tendency that represents the most frequently occurring value or category in the distribution.

negative correlation   Occurs when two variables move in opposite directions; also known as an *inverse relationship*.

nominal measurement   A level of measurement for categorical variables. It is the lowest level of measurement.

nondirectional hypothesis   A hypothesis in which no specific direction is stated; the hypothesis simply states that there will be a difference/relationship between variables.

nonexperimental design   A type of design used to *describe, test relationships*, or *compare,* but not to determine cause and effect.

nonprobability sampling   A method of nonrandomly selecting subjects for a sample who are available to the investigator. Convenience, quota, and snowballing are nonprobability sampling methods.

null hypothesis   A declarative statement that indicates that there is not a relationship or an effect between two or more variables; also known as the *statistical hypothesis*.

operational definition   The definition of a variable that describes exactly how the variable will be measured.

ordinal measurement   A level of measurement for categorical variables, which is higher than nominal level because there is a rank order.

outcomes research   The study of how to achieve outcomes that matter to patients.

p value   The probability value associated with a test statistic. The smaller the p value (generally <.05), the more confidence there is that the difference in findings were not due to chance.

paradata   Data that is transparently captured that assists in evaluating the usability of Web-administered tools. Paradata can be termed as server side, which are data related to global aspects of instrument usage, or client side, which are data related to individual behavior use patterns.

phenomenology   A type of qualitative study that focuses on the "lived experience" of participants.

population   A population consists of all the people, objects, units, or events of a clearly defined group that meet the specific criteria under investigation.

positive correlation   Occurs when the values of both variables move together in the same direction.

power   The ability to find a difference or association when one actually exists.

primary source   A research article that reports the methods and results of an original research study performed by the authors of the study.

probability sampling   A method of randomly selecting cases, objects, or units by using either simple random, stratified random, proportionate stratified random, systematic, or cluster sampling from a population.

probability   How likely it is that a particular outcome will randomly occur.

program of research   When one study builds upon the next, developing a body of knowledge on one topic, rather than several studies conducted on an assortment of unrelated topics.

proportional stratified sample   A sampling strategy used to maintain the same proportion or percentage of subjects within each category, assuring that each grouping is equally represented in the study.

prospective design   A time element of research design. The research question is answered by following the subjects forward in time to see if the outcome of interest occurs, also known as a *cohort design.*

qualitative research   Research that explores the content, meaning, and nature of phenomenon using such techniques as interviewing and observation.

quality improvement   An internal process by which processes and outcomes of practice are evaluated for quick intervention in an organization; also called *performance improvement.*

quantitative research   Research that investigates scientific questions with tools that produce statistical measurements.

quasiexperimental design   A type of experimental design that lacks randomization; also known as a *nonrandomized trial.*

quota sampling   A nonrandom method of assigning subjects to the sample; based on a set number or percentage (quota) of a sample characteristic.

random assignment   A method of assignment that ensures that each study participant has an equal chance of being assigned to the various study groups, also known as *randomization.*

random sampling   Probability sampling that uses a method such as a random number generator to assure that each individual has an equal chance of being selected.

range   The range of the variable describes the difference between the maximum and minimum values.

ratio measurement   The highest level of measurement. It differs from interval only in that it has a meaningful zero.

refereed journal   Journals with rigorous standards for screening manuscripts prior to publication. Peer reviewers make a recommendation to the editor of the journal on whether the journal should publish the manuscript, or if changes need to be made prior to publication. Nonrefereed publications, however, are not peer reviewed.

regression analysis   A statistical test that allows the researcher to examine the effect of multiple independent variables on a single dependent variable.

reliability   In terms of instruments, the stability—or trustworthiness—of a measure.

Repeated Measures ANOVA   A statistical test used to examine the differences in an outcome variable at the interval/ratio level among one group with the outcome variable measured at multiple points over time.

replication research   The deliberate repetition of research procedures in a second investigation for the purpose of determining if earlier results can be repeated.

research   A systematic investigation designed to contribute to generalizable knowledge.

research hypothesis   A declarative statement that indicates there is a relationship between two or more variables and suggests an answer to the related research question.

research proposal   A written plan describing all of the elements of a study, including the background, theory, and methodology.

research protocol   A document that details each step required to conduct the study.

research question   An interrogative statement that frames a question about the relationship or effect of one variable on another in a specific population. Research questions can be descriptive (asking about the characteristics of a population), correlational (asking about the relationship between two or more variables), intervention (asking about the effect of one variable on others), or meaning/essence (asking about the experience of a phenomenon as it is lived by specific individuals).

retrospective design   A time element of research design. The dependent variable is in the present and the question is answered by looking back in time for presumed causes. Often used for chart review studies.

sample   A selected subset of the target population.

sampling frame   A list of all the persons (units, cases) in the population from which the sample is drawn.

sampling plan   A plan of action for participant selection or recruitment that includes sampling method, sample size, and procedures for recruitment.

scale   A form of self-report tool used in nursing and psychological research that is often used to elicit responses about attitudes, traits, or intensity of symptoms.

scholarly publication   A term that is often used to refer to a manuscript published in a refereed journal.

secondary source   Articles written to review a topic or summarize the findings of other authors and researchers.

significance level   The level of certainty the researcher determines is necessary to conclude there is statistical significance.

simple random sampling   A sampling method that provides an equal chance (probability) of all persons (units, cases) to be selected for sample.

skip pattern   An electronic feature that allows for automatic skipping over irrelevant questions.

snowball sampling   A nonprobability sampling method that asks current sample members to identify additional potential participants, also known as *network sampling*.

social media   A mode of communication that is Internet based and allows participants to interact with the medium and/or users of the medium.

stakeholder   A person or organization who holds a special interest in the results of a project.

standard deviation   Describes the average distance the values are from the variable's center.

statistical hypothesis   A declarative statement that indicates that there is not a relationship or an effect between two or more variables; also known as the *null hypothesis*.

statistical significance   The difference observed between two samples is large enough so that it is not simply due to chance (p < alpha).

stratified random sampling   A sampling method that divides the sampling frame into categories or groups prior to conducting the random sample assignment within each group.

student t-test   A statistical test used to determine if there is a difference in the average value of a variable in two samples when the outcome variable is at the interval or ratio level.

survey study   A type of descriptive study often used to seek opinions, attitudes, health care needs, knowledge deficits, and barriers and facilitators to practice, among other things.

systematic sampling   A sampling method in which a set sampling interval of every k^{th} (e.g., 3rd or 4th) subject is selected.

test/retest reliability   A form of reliability that ensures that the measure works well or is stable on repeated administrations.

theoretical definition   An abstract definition of a concept, also known as the *conceptual definition*.

translation research   The study of how to get scientific discoveries into practice applications.

trustworthiness   The extent to which the researcher has demonstrated that the results of the study are an accurate reflection of the participants' experiences.

Type I error   An error that is committed when the null hypothesis is accepted as false when it is actually true.

Type II error   An error that is committed when the null hypothesis is accepted as true when it is actually false.

validity   In terms of instruments, the degree to which an instrument measures what it intends to measure.

variable   A characteristic that can have more than one value—that is, it varies.

vulnerable subject   One who demonstrates limited capacity or freedom to participate or to decline to participate in research.

worldview   The principles and beliefs that guide how you approach life.

Index

D

H

J–K

L

Q

R